Understanding Work-Related Musculoskeletal Disorders

A comprehensive guide to tackle Work-Related Musculoskeletal Issues for professionals

DR. PINKY DUTTA

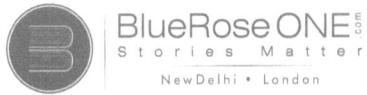

BLUEROSE PUBLISHERS
India | U.K.

Copyright © Dr. Pinky Dutta 2024

All rights reserved by author. No part of this publication may be reproduced, stored in a retrieval system or transmitted in any form or by any means, electronic, mechanical, photocopying, recording or otherwise, without the prior permission of the author. Although every precaution has been taken to verify the accuracy of the information contained herein, the publisher assumes no responsibility for any errors or omissions. No liability is assumed for damages that may result from the use of information contained within.

BlueRose Publishers takes no responsibility for any damages, losses, or liabilities that may arise from the use or misuse of the information, products, or services provided in this publication.

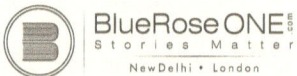

For permissions requests or inquiries regarding this publication, please contact:

BLUEROSE PUBLISHERS
www.BlueRoseONE.com
info@bluerosepublishers.com
+91 8882 898 898
+4407342408967

ISBN: 978-93-6261-155-0

Cover design: Suruchi
Typesetting: Rohit

First Edition: June 2024

Preface

Work-related musculoskeletal disorders (WRMSDs) are a major public health problem, affecting millions of workers worldwide. WRMSDs can cause pain, discomfort, and disability, and can lead to lost productivity and increased healthcare costs. This pocket book is designed to provide a comprehensive overview of WRMSDs, including their causes, prevention, and management. It is written for a wide audience, including workers, employers, healthcare professionals, and policymakers. I am particularly pleased to have written this book as an Associate Professor in the Garden City College of Physiotherapy. In my role as a teacher and researcher, I have seen firsthand the impact that WRMSDs can have on workers' lives. I am passionate about helping people prevent and manage these disorders, and I hope that this book will make a valuable contribution to this effort.

The book is divided into five chapters. Chapter 1 provides an introduction to WRMSDs, including their definition, epidemiology, and risk factors. Chapter 2 discusses ergonomics and workplace design, and how these principles can be used to reduce the risk of WRMSDs. Chapter 3 reviews common occupation-related MSDs and their management. Chapter 4 discusses workplace prevention and management strategies for WRMSDs. Chapter 5 covers legal and ethical considerations related to WRMSDs.

I would like to acknowledge the many people who have contributed to this book. First and foremost, I would like to thank my colleagues and students at the Garden City College of Physiotherapy for their support and encouragement. I would also like to thank my family and friends for their patience and understanding. I hope that this book will be a valuable resource for all those who are interested in learning more about WRMSDs and how to prevent and manage them. In addition to the above, I would like to add a few more thoughts on the importance of this book. WRMSDs are a major cause of absenteeism and disability, and they can have a significant impact on workers' quality of life. However, many WRMSDs are preventable. By understanding the causes of WRMSDs and taking steps to reduce risk factors, workers can protect themselves from these disorders. This book provides a concise and easy-to-understand overview of WRMSDs, including their causes, prevention, and management. It is written in a clear and engaging style, and it is appropriate for a wide audience.

I believe that this book can make a significant contribution to the prevention and management of WRMSDs. I encourage all workers, employers, healthcare professionals, and policymakers to read this book and learn more about this important topic.

Contents

1. Introduction to Work Related Musculoskeletal Disorders (WRMSD) 1
2. Ergonomics And Workplace Design 51
3. Common Occupation Related MSDs And Their Management 117
4. Workplace Prevention And Management Strategies 229
5. Legal And Ethical Considerations 272

Chapter 1:

Introduction to Work Related Musculoskeletal Disorders (WRMSD)

Introduction

Musculoskeletal disorders (MSDs) are a diverse group of medical conditions that affect the muscles, bones, tendons, ligaments, and other supportive structures of the body [1]. These disorders can cause pain, discomfort, and limitations in movement, often impacting a person's ability to perform daily activities and work tasks. MSDs can affect people of all ages and backgrounds and are a significant cause of disability and healthcare utilization worldwide [2]. Work related Musculoskeletal Disorders (WRMSD or WMSD) refer to the injuries to bones and muscles due to repetitive stress from occupational activities. This comprises about 50% of the non-fatal occupational injury cases [1,3].

The use of observational methodologies, tools, and checklists is the foundation of the risk evaluation and management process for occupational risk factors implicated in the etiopathogenesis of WMSDs, such as uncomfortable postures, repetitive motions, manual handling of heavy weights, and extended computer work. For instance, Directive 90/269/EEC specifies the technical requirements of the International Organisation for Standardisation (ISO) 11,228 series as the reference approach in the risk assessment of human handling of high loads [1,2]. These standards employ various widely recognized analysis techniques. However, it should be highlighted that a thorough examination more ISO ergonomics standards in terms of biomechanical stress assessment has uncovered several important concerns. Additionally, when this sort of risk is linked to additional occupational risk factors, particularly when a situation of continuous computer use arises, the assessment of difficult poses is frequently conducted [2]. Directive 90/270/EEC concerning risk connected with electronic screen (like computers) usage at the workplace underlined that working using a screen for more than 20 hours per week indicates a serious risk condition that requires the activation of a medical surveillance system in this respect. Typically, interviews based on a checklist or self-administered questionnaires are used to determine the duration of the working period where looking at an electronic screen or monitor is required. Again, occupations involving lifting of heavy objects, sudden application of high-force, limited tasks or performing a job involving limited movements, static muscle loads, tasks requiring involvement of cognitive demands, and working at undesirable temperatures, can bring stress to the musculoskeletal system and prolong occurrence can have poor prognosis in terms of development of disorders [3]. Therefore, it is essential that the development and subsequent implementation of effective preventative strategies are based on precise, trustworthy, and high-quality quantitative data that highlights the true scope of the prevalence of WMSD [4].

Although forceful or repeated tasks sometimes cause injuries to many body regions at once, upper limb WMSDs constitute the fastest-growing subset of occupational illnesses. Repetitive strain injuries is a phrase used to describe illnesses brought on by repetitive motions, uncomfortable postures, force, and/or associated risk factors rather than a specific diagnosis. The phrase cumulative trauma disorder is gaining favour in the US. The phrase "cervicobrachial syndrome" was widely used in Scandinavia and Japan. The World Health Organisation accepts the phrase "work-related" to cover multiple reasons, however, some detractors disapprove due to the term's etiologic connotation. Thus, WMSD does appear to be a suitable name for multifactorial changes to the muscle-tendon unit that can be initiated or made worse by peripheral neurons and the vascular system by using the upper limbs physically and/or repeatedly [5].

Common musculoskeletal issues at work

Although diverse terminologies and methodological issues have hampered critical scientific exchange within the medical profession, there has been significant progress in recent years regarding case definitions applicable in certain circumstances [6].

For instance, in the Palmar-plantar syndrome, the median nerve becomes squeezed in the channel to the wrist that is delineated by the flexor tendons, the longitudinal carpal ligament, and the carpal bones, resulting in carpal tunnel syndrome, which is most often diagnosed of the WMSDs [5,6]. Chronic illnesses (such as gout, hypothyroidism, and diabetes mellitus), as well as rheumatic diseases, menopause, pregnancy, and oestrogen usage, are among the medical factors linked to CTS. A risk factor for inflammatory arthritis, diabetes, as well as untreated hypothyroidism, was observed. However, the information was unclear for other non-occupational illnesses. Congenital malformations, non-occupational activities, small wrist size, and trauma must all be taken into account. However, it's important to remember that the presence of a non-occupational risk factor doesn't always rule out a potential workplace contribution [7].

Normal symptoms of carpal tunnel syndrome include nocturnal discomfort, weakness, and paresthesias. According to conventional wisdom [4,5], tingling in the median nerve distribution in conjunction with a positive Tinel's sign (inducing paresthesias by tapping the wrist in the median nerve) and Phalen's manoeuvre (reproducing symptoms through maximum wrist flexion) was indicative of the diagnosis, and nerve conduction studies are required to confirm the diagnosis [5]. Tinel's sign is a medical diagnostic test used to assess nerve irritation or injury, particularly in cases of nerve compression or entrapment. The test is named after French neurologist Jules Tinel, who first described it. It is commonly used to evaluate conditions like carpal tunnel syndrome and other nerve-related disorders. During a Tinel's sign test, a physiotherapist can lightly tap or tap along the path of a specific nerve with their fingers or a reflex hammer [6]. If the nerve is irritated or compressed, the patient may experience a tingling sensation or "pins and needles" feeling radiating along the nerve's distribution, typically into the extremities. For instance, in the case of carpal tunnel syndrome, the median nerve passing through the wrist can become compressed, leading to symptoms like pain, numbness, and tingling in the thumb, index finger, middle finger, and half of the ring finger [7]. Physiotherapists use multiple tests and consider other clinical information to make more specific diagnoses. Figure 1 shows the Tinel's sign. When a Tinel's sign test is performed by tapping lightly over the wrist area where the median nerve travels, a positive result might elicit the characteristic tingling sensation along the nerve's path. It's important to note that while a positive Tinel's sign can suggest nerve irritation or compression, it is just one component of a comprehensive clinical evaluation [4,5].

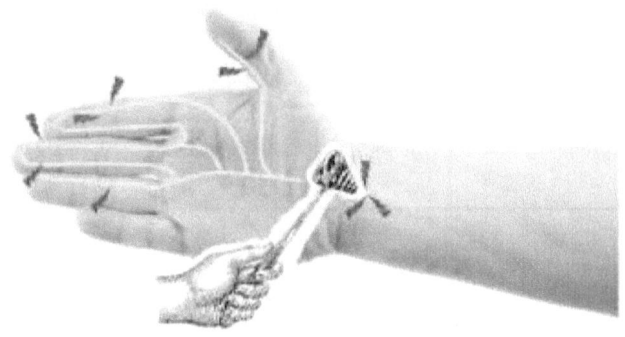

Figure 1: Tinel's sign

Negative results from testing should not be taken to mean that the diagnosis has been ruled out because nerve conduction problems sometimes do not manifest until late into the process of entrapment. Additionally, there is very little consistency between the electrodiagnostic results of CTS and symptom questionnaires, physical examination techniques, and those results. In some circumstances, noninvasive testing like high-resolution sonography or magnetic resonance imaging may be helpful [8].

Table 1: Common risk variables for a selection of musculoskeletal illnesses caused by labour from whose definitions have been generated

Disorder	Case definition	Surveillance Criteria	Risk factors
The wrist's tenosynovitis	Extensor or flexor tendon sheath inflammation at the wrist	Pain is reproduced by resisting vigorous movement of the injured tendons while the forearm is stabilised and localised to the wrist's afflicted tendon sheaths.	wrist repeatedly moving out of neutral position; force, vibration, and mechanical stress
Wrist de Quervain's disease	Extensor pollicis brevis the adductor pollicis longus' initial extensor compartment is painfully swollen.	Pain that is localised to the radial styloid and is accompanied by tenderness and edema in the first extensor compartment. This pain may either be replicated by resisting thumb extension or by a positive Finkelstein test.	Thumb overuse, and ulnar or radial wrist deviation

Elbow and forearm lateral epicondylitis	a lesion at the lateral epicondyle at the humerus's common extensor origin that results in the symptoms listed in the criterion	Lateral epicondylar discomfort, epicondylar soreness, and pain when the wrist is extended against resistance	Long-term hammer usage, repetitive forearm pronation, and supination, strong wrist extension, or gripping with an extended arm

| Neck and Shoulder tendinitis | symptoms of rotator cuff and biceps tendon inflammation or deterioration | Resisted active motions (abduction of the supraspinatus, external rotation for the infraspinatus, teres minor, and internal rotation of the subscapularis) and soreness in the deltoid area are all symptoms of rotator cuff problems. Biceps: a history of anterior shoulder discomfort, pain with vigorous elbow flexion against resistance, or pain with supination of the forearm [10]. | using one's arm repeatedly in abduction and flexion or raising it; force |

Syndrome of the thoracic outlet	a collection of symptoms and warning signals in the hand or arm brought on by the thoracic outlet compressing the neurovascular bundle	None established; in UK medical practise, an extremely unusual disease.	Reaching above shoulder level repeatedly, holding weights out to the side for an extended period of time, wearing a rucksack, or bracing shoulders when carrying a cargo
Achilles tendinitis	Pain and inflammation of the Achilles tendon	Pain and tenderness along the Achilles tendon, swelling, difficulty walking or running	Age, overuse, poor footwear, tight calf muscles
Patellofemoral pain syndrome	Pain in front of the knee, often worse with activities that involve kneeling or squatting	Pain and tenderness in front of the knee, crepitus (a crackling sound) when the knee is moved, weakness of the quadriceps muscles	Age, female sex, obesity, alignment problems of the knee
Shin splints	Pain along the inner or outer edge of the shinbone	Pain and tenderness along the shinbone, worse with exercise	Overuse, poor footwear, flat feet

Plantar fasciitis	Pain in the heel or arch of the foot	Pain and tenderness in the heel or arch of the foot, worse in the morning or after prolonged standing	Age, obesity, flat feet, excessive pronation of the foot
Stress fracture	A small crack in the bone	Pain in the bone that worsens with activity, swelling, bruising	Overuse, poor training technique, fatigue
Osteoarthritis	Degeneration of the cartilage in a joint	Pain, stiffness, swelling, decreased range of motion	Age, obesity, previous injury, repetitive stress
Rheumatoid arthritis	Autoimmune disease that causes inflammation of the joints	Pain, stiffness, swelling, redness, warmth of the joints, decreased range of motion	Age, family history, smoking

In musculoskeletal disorders, anatomical structures like muscles, ligaments, tendons, joints, peripheral nerves, and other structures are all affected by a variety of inflammatory and degenerative pathology, and the blood vessels are also affected [11]. Among them are clinical syndromes like tendon inflammations and related illnesses (tenosynovitis, epicondylitis, bursitis), compression of nerves problems (carpal tunnel syndrome, sciatica), or osteoarthrosis, in addition to less well-defined conditions like myalgia, low back pain, and other regional pain syndromes not associated with known pathology [6].

Lower back, neck, shoulder, forearm, and hand are the body parts most frequently affected, however recently, attention has been focused more on the lower extremities [7].

Musculoskeletal diseases (MSDs) are common in many nations and have a significant financial and quality of life effect. Despite not being specifically connected to employment, they account for a sizable fraction of all job-related illnesses that have been reported and/or are eligible for compensation in many nations. It is challenging to get precise information about the prevalence and incidence of musculoskeletal illnesses, and it is even more challenging to compare national figures [8].

Certain sectors and vocations have rates of MSDs that are as much as three to four times greater than the average. Nursing homes, air travel, mining, food processing, food tanning, heavy and light manufacturing (vehicles, furniture, appliances, electronic devices, textiles, clothes, and shoes), and nursing facilities are some of the high-risk industries [5]. The prevalence of upper extremity musculoskeletal problems is also quite high in manual labor-intensive jobs like office work, postal delivery, cleaning, industrial inspection, and packing. Truck drivers, warehouse workers, airline baggage handlers, building trades, nurses, nursing assistants, and other patient-care employees, as well as drivers of cranes and other heavy vehicles, are more likely than the general population to experience back and lower limb diseases [9].

Insufficient recovery time, heavy lifting and strenuous manual labour, non-neutral body positions (either dynamic or static), mechanical pressure concentrations, segmental or whole-body vibration, local or whole-body exposure to cold, and any of these in combination are among the physical job features which are frequently cited as risk factors over MSDs, based on both experimental science and epidemiologic investigations [10].

One of the most prevalent issues at work is musculoskeletal diseases (MSDs). Muscle, joint, tendon, and nerve disorders (MSDs) can affect the neck, upper limbs, and back, among other body areas. Work-associated musculoskeletal conditions (WMSDs) are thought to be the primary cause of work-related injuries, lower quality of life, changing occupations, and rising medical costs owing to disability [11].

People work long hours in front of computers in various professions like engineering, administration jobs, and design to name a few. Most of the time, office workers need to sit for 8 to 12 hours at a stretch in their offices. Computer use has grown at work, and this has led to symptoms of MSDs, which are more common than 50% of the time, notably throughout the upper extremities as well as the lower back. Office employees frequently have neck, shoulder, and lower back pain or discomfort from MSDs as a result of their prolonged sitting positions. MSDs are common around the world and can have both negative socioeconomic and individual effects [12].

Fast-paced work, uncomfortable postures, extended sitting, and highly repetitive activities are all associated with MSDs and pain/discomfort at work. Additionally, unhealthy and insufficient working conditions can result in MSDs, negatively impact people's welfare and wellbeing, and decrease productivity [13].

1.2 Classification

Since it has been researched for more than a century, the classification from musculoskeletal disorders (MSDs), known as disorders of tendinous, muscular, and articular origin, remains significant in the medical community. The grouping of MSDs includes a wide range of conditions, including tendonitis, tendinosis, arthrosis, and degenerative joint lesions that can be caused by tendon compression [14].

The "onset" of the injury's occurrence, whether abrupt or recurring, determines the most common clinical classification. Its practical use in recognizing some injuries, meanwhile, is very simple and causes confusion due to neurological abnormalities, especially when it comes to acute damage to wounded tissues or progressive injuries. Five injury classifications were upgraded in sports during the past ten years to help with the MSD classification.

According to a pathophysiological setting, both acute and chronic inflammatory processes contribute to the development of all MSDs [15].

Table 2. Modified classification criteria based on tissue changes and injury pathophysiology

Classification	Description	Clinical Signs	Cytokine	Duration Time	Outcomes
Acute Inflammation	Small blood vessels expand. increased permeability of microvessels. Leukocyte migration: From 24 to 48 hours following injury, macrophages gradually replace the neutrophils that predominate during the first 6 to 24 hours.	Blush fever edema pain	TNF, IL-1, IL-6, and IL-17 Bradykinin, Prostaglandins, and Reactive Oxygen Species	24–48 h	- complete healing - cell function that is reversible - Progressive chronic inflammation and consequently cell death.

Transition Period	Features of chronic and acute inflammation can be observed between 48 hours and 7 days. The period during which it is unclear whether an injury is chronic or acute is known as the transitional phase.				
Chronic Inflammation	- a prolonged reaction that begins 48 hours after an injury and lasts over weeks or months. In the current phase, various combinations of tissue injury, inflammation, and healing efforts coexist. - Macrophages or T lymphocytes are the predominate cells in the majority of chronic inflammatory responses.	suffering atrophy	IL-12 INF IL-17	≥7 days	− Loss of function, fibrosis, and maybe even tissue collapse might happen. Neuropathic pain, granulation tissue, neural fibrosis, anxiety, and depression

In the acute stage of the inflammation, if the inflammatory process cannot eliminate tissue injury or rejuvenate new tissue Such overburden will accelerate the inflammatory process, causing the inflammation to become chronic. WRMSDs can be categorized by the International Labour Standards (ILO) as either occupational illnesses with a code or occupational accidents. The International Classification of Diseases (ICD) defines a work-aggravated disease as any other damage that is not included in these two categories. ICD assigns a code for classification to categories related to MSDs, although this code is not appropriate for usage in a clinical treatment context [16].

According to the National Institute for Occupational Safety and Health (NIOSH) classification, the risk factors that are acknowledged as occupational can be considered a method of occurrence of WRMSD injuries. However, in the context of the workplace, the significance of Bernard and colleagues' classification is limited to identifying the risk factors that might result in occupational disorders acknowledged by ILO. It does not, however, provide data that explains the pathophysiological mechanism of injuries. Despite the absence of information, Bernard's classification was frequently used in the context of worker safety and health and the field of work ergonomics [17].

According to the European Agency of Safety and Health during Work (EU-OSHA), "WRMSDs" are disorders that are primarily brought on by or made worse by work and the surroundings in which it is conducted. However, despite the fact that this classification is important in the case of medico-legal situations, it seldom applies in actual physiotherapy practice [18].

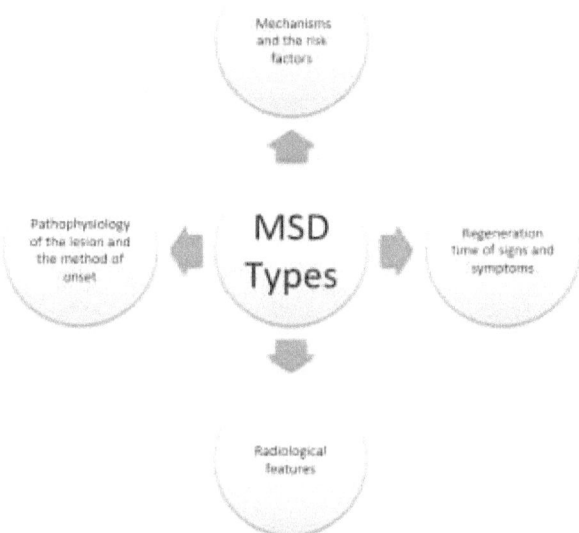

Figure 2: Musculoskeletal Disorder (MSD) has been classified according to the pathophysiology of the lesion and the method of onset, mechanisms and the risk factors, the regeneration time of signs and symptoms and radiological features.

Figure 2 has been explained in detail in the following section.

Table 3 lists the previously established scale grades (MSD-0 to MSD-3) in accordance with the forensic medicine standards, tying them to the causes of tissue injury and the risk factors discovered in the workplace. The risk variables in this evaluation were broken down into four categories: operational (risks linked with working duties), ergonomic (primarily variables related to physical biomechanics of movement), and individual (risks that involve bone misalignments as well as muscle imbalances) [19].

Table 3. Criteria based on the pathophysiology of the lesion and the method of onset

Classification	Criterion			
MSD Type	Onset Mode	Inflammation	Tissue	Results of Tissue Regeneration
0	Late	Acute	Healthy	Regeneration of the whole tissue (regeneration without permanent cellular alterations)
1	Sudden	Acute	Healthy	fully regenerating tissue without fibrosis
2	Sudden	Chronic	Healthy or Altered	Cell death, fibrosis, and persistent, increasing inflammation
3	Gradual	Chronic	Altered	granulation of tissue, fibrosis, and loss of function neural fibrosis and neuropathic pain

Table 4 displays the relationships between the MSD scales 0–3 as well as clinical symptoms such as pain (measured using the visual analogical pain scale), injury zone, as well as therapy (discussed in the literature of internal medicine, orthopaedics, physiatry, and medical semiology), which are also used in other international classifications. In this table, the classification criteria are categorized based on the MSD (Musculoskeletal Disorder) Type, Onset Mode, Mechanical Action, Tissue Integrity and Tissue Injury Mechanism, and Risk Factor. Each classification is associated with specific injury mechanisms and patterns, helping to understand the nature of the injuries, how they occur, and the factors contributing to their occurrence. The table highlights the continuum of injury types, from late tissue damage caused by the manageable effort to sudden injuries due to external trauma or excessive effort. It also underscores the distinction between mechanical actions, tissue integrity, and inflammatory mechanisms that contribute to different injury patterns. Additionally, the table indicates the relevant risk factors for each injury classification, ranging from personal and physical factors to operational and ergonomic considerations. This classification framework is valuable for identifying, preventing, and managing various types of injuries in different contexts. It aids in designing effective strategies for injury prevention, workplace ergonomics, and overall health and safety.

Table 4: Classification of injuries based on their mechanisms and the risk factors that come with each activity

Classification		Criterion		
		Mechanism/Risk Factors		
MSD Type	Onset Mode	Mechanical Action	Tissue Integrity and Tissue Injury Mechanism	Risk Factor
0	Late	tissue damage brought on by a manageable effort	change in homeostasis accompanied by a minor inflammatory reaction	Absent
1	Sudden	−Excessive effort-related tissue damage from external direct trauma	traumatising, causing a flare-up of severe inflammation within healthy tissue	Operationally Physical
2	Sudden	Direct external injury Tissue damage brought on by excessive effort	an abrupt flare-up of inflammation in tissue that has already been injured or inflamed but hasn't totally recovered.	.personal physical operationally ergonomic

3	Gradual	Injury to inflammatory and fibrous tissue that might happen with minimal effort	Chronic inflammation is maintained by recurrent bouts of inflammation over non-regenerating tissue.	Individual physical operational ergonomic

MSD Type 0 is characterized as "Late" onset, where individuals experience mild discomfort that exacerbates with activity and subsides naturally within 48 hours. The anatomical involvement pertains to "Muscles, Ligaments, and Tendons." There's no specified need for treatment or rehabilitation. MSD Type 1 corresponds to a "Sudden" onset with severe pain following an accident, intensifying over time regardless of incapacitation. Symptoms include muscular contractures, discomfort upon palpation, potential generalization, local swelling, hyperemia, hematomas, pain during movement, and restricted range of motion. Affected anatomical areas encompass "Joints, Ligaments/Tendons, Muscles, and Bones." Both treatment and rehabilitation are deemed necessary. MSD Type 2 also exhibits a "Sudden" onset, characterized by acute inflammation worsening with movement and lasting for days or weeks, possibly leading to incapacitation. Anxiety due to moderate to severe pain restricts range of motion during palpation or free movement. Similar anatomical areas are affected: "Joints, Muscles, Ligaments/Tendons, and Bones." Treatment and rehabilitation are both indicated. MSD Type 3 presents a "Gradual" onset involving continual functional loss and moderate to mild, chronic inflammatory discomfort. This condition is task-related, necessitating regular painkiller use for management. It often connects with paraesthesia (abnormal sensations) and worsens during activity but improves with rest.

The affected anatomical areas are again "Joints, Muscles, Ligaments/Tendons, and Bones." Treatment and rehabilitation are recommended.

Table 5: Classification based on the criteria for establishing the regeneration time of signs and symptoms

Classification		Criterion			
		Clinical	Anatomical	Treatment	
MSD Type	Onset mode	Signs and symptoms	Injury zone	Rest	Rehabilitation
0	Late	Mild discomfort that becomes worse with activity and goes away spontaneously lasting up to 48 hours.	Muscles Ligaments and tendons	No need	No need

| 1 | Sudden | severe pain from the time of the accident that gets worse with time, whether it's incapacitating or not. Muscular contracture, discomfort on severe palpation, occasionally generalised, local oedema, hyperemia, the existence of a hematoma, pain when moving, and a reduced range of motion are some of the symptoms that may be present. | Joints, Ligaments/Tendons, Muscles, and Bones | Need | Need |

| 2 | Sudden | Acute, ongoing inflammation that worsens with movement can last for days or weeks and is potentially incapacitating. The range of motion is reduced because of anxiety when in moderate to severe pain while palpation or free movement. | Joints, Muscles, Ligaments/Tendons, and Bones | Need | Need |

3	Gradual	Continual loss of function and moderate to mild chronic inflammatory discomfort. Task-related and requires the regular usage of painkillers to manage. It is frequently linked to paraesthesia and can get worse during task movement and get better with rest.	Joints, Muscles, Ligaments/Tendons, and Bones	Need	Need

Table 6 displays the correlation between radiological results and the MSD 0-3 scale. In a study, the findings are laid out descriptively and narratively, with the reference to earlier classifications acknowledged in the specialty literature [20].

Table 6: Classification of MSDs based on radiological features

Classification		Criterion
MSD Type	Onset Mode	Radiology/Complementary Examinations (USG/RM)
0	Late	Slight exudate oedema.
1	Sudden	High-resolution MRI is often positive for fibre breaking when necessary. an intramuscular haemorrhage. Exudate (oedema). when a high-resolution MRI detects a partial fibre break. Intramuscular haemorrhage with thin, disorganised fibres surrounded by haemorrhage and peripheral fluid. When the muscle fibres completely discontinue, there is a haemorrhage, and the muscles in the extremities retract. MRI and USG are comparable.
2	Sudden	Positive when the fibres are dislocated, partially or completely ruptured, sometimes with considerable retraction. It could be oedematous and hemorrhagic. Haematoma and peri-fascial fluid are present around disorganised, thin tendon fibres that are undergoing bone remodelling and tendon calcification processes.On an MRI after a total rupture, the following findings are noted: "Complete discontinuity the muscle fibres, haematoma, as well as retraction the muscular extremities. MRI and USG are comparable.

| 3 | Gradual | positive for a degenerative condition, frequently accompanied with atrophy, dysplasia, and some ligamentous retraction. Oedema, haematoma, bone remodelling, and laborious calcification processes are possible. |

Common Risk Factors and Causes

Injury or malfunction of the tissues, nerves, tendons, ligaments, bones, cartilages, or spinal discs are referred to as musculoskeletal diseases. Sprains, strains, rips, stiffness, discomfort, carpal tunnel syndrome, hernias, or connective tissue injuries to the aforementioned structures are all examples of musculoskeletal illnesses. Several epidemiological studies have shown evidence of a causal association between physical exertion while at work and, in accordance with the National Institute of Occupational Health and Safety (NIOSH), Musculoskeletal conditions at work (WMSD). WMSD has been linked to a number of causes, including extended sitting and standing, awkward or persistent postures, repetitive movements, and excessive force [21].

More than 600,000 people in the US alone have WMSD, which requires days of absence from work every year. Additionally, WMSD is the priciest type of job disability. Different risk factors apply to various types of WMSD, such as low back WMSD, carpal tunnel syndrome, tendinitis in epicondylitis, etc. It is challenging for single research to meet all requirements for establishing a causal link between risk variables and WMSD. Therefore, it is crucial to combine and analyze data from the research done on the etiologies of various forms of WMSD. Risk factors and the strength of the evidence supporting their connection to each WMSD may then be assessed [22].

Neck

Psychosocial variables, smoking, female gender, uncomfortable postures, and co-morbidities were the key risk factors shown to have sufficient evidence proving their causal association with neck WMSD. Awkward postures were listed as a risk factor for the onset of neck WMSD in the NIOSH report. However, despite the fact that the NIOSH study said that repetitive and vigorous labour had adequate evidence to establish their status as risk factors of WMSD [23].

Shoulder

Heavy physical labour and psychosocial variables were the key risk factors that had solid evidence supporting a causal link with shoulder WMSD.

Wrist/hand

Computer use, strenuous physical labour, awkward posture, repetitive motions, elevated BMI, advanced age, and female gender were the key risk variables identified as having probable proof supporting their causal link with wrist/hand WMSD. According to the NIOSH analysis, computer use, strenuous physical activity, and vibration were risk factors in the onset of wrist and hand discomfort. However, despite the NIOSH review's identification of vibration as a distinct risk factor for hand/wrist WMSD [24].

Lower back

Heavy physical work, uncomfortable postures, lifting, psychosocial variables, higher BMI, and younger age were the key risk factors that had sufficient evidence to establish their causal link with low back WMSD. Uncomfortable working positions, lifting, or whole-body vibration were listed as risk factors in the NIOSH report for the emergence of low back WMSD [25].

Hip

Heavy physical labour and lifting were the key risk variables that had solid evidence pointing to a link between them and hip WMSD [24,25].

Knee

Mis-align postures, pulling repetition, and co-morbidities were the key risk variables with sufficient evidence to suggest their causal link with knee WMSD. The analysis and modification of the workplace to lower knee WMSD should take into account the risk variables that were determined to have adequate evidence [26].

Certain sectors and vocations have rates of MSDs that are as much as three to four times greater than the average. Nursing homes, air travel, mining, food processing, food tanning, heavy and light manufacturing (vehicles, furniture, appliances, electronic devices, textiles, clothes, and shoes), and nursing facilities are some of the high-risk industries [25]. The prevalence of upper extremity musculoskeletal problems is also quite high in manual labor-intensive jobs like office work, postal delivery, cleaning, industrial inspection, and packing. Truck drivers, workers in warehouses, airline baggage handlers, building trades, nurses, nursing assistants, and other patient-care employees, as well as drivers of cranes and other heavy vehicles, are more likely than the general population to experience back and lower limb diseases [27]. Insufficient recovery time, heavy lifting and strenuous manual labour, non-neutral body positions (either dynamic or static), mechanical pressure concentrations, segmental or whole-body vibration, local or whole-body exposure to cold, and any of these in combination are among the physical job features which are frequently cited as risk factors over MSDs, based on both experimental science and epidemiologic investigations [28].

High background rate, and several risk factors

MSDs have a variety of risk factors, including occupational and non-occupational, like the majority of chronic illnesses.

In addition to the responsibilities of the workplace, activities like housekeeping and sports can put physical strain on the musculoskeletal structures. Systemic illnesses such as rheumatoid arthritis, gout, lupus, and diabetes have an impact on the musculoskeletal and peripheral nerve tissues. Age, gender, financial level, and ethnicity all affect risk differently. Obesity, smoking, muscle strength, and other features of job ability are some other hypothesized risk factors [29].

The NRC/IOM panel and the majority of writers agreed that these illnesses had a complex aetiology in the general population. Not everyone who has an MSD has ergonomic workplace exposure, and not everyone who is exposed at work experiences an MSD. The term "work-related disorders" is more suitable here [90], as opposed to "occupational disorders" when a single element is both required and sufficient to induce the disease (for example, mesothelioma brought on by asbestos exposure) [28-30].

Some have suggested that occupational variables cannot fully explain the burden of musculoskeletal illness because of the prevalence of these disorders in the general population and the numerous non-occupational risk factors. This makes no sense at all. One risk factor's presence does not rule out another. To what degree people may be safeguarded against preventable dangers at work is not the same topic as whether occupational variables contribute to few or many MSDs for the general population [28,30,31].

Epidemiology and Prevalence

Epidemiology

Musculoskeletal problems are thought to affect 1.71 billion individuals globally, making them the primary cause of disability and misery. In 160 of the 204 nations studied, low back pain was the leading cause of disability. Muscle, tendon, ligament, joint, and bone illnesses and injuries are together referred to as "musculoskeletal disorders" (MSDs) [32].

MSDs might cause discomfort and impairment by affecting the back, the cervical area, as well as the upper and lower extremities. In 2017, there was some inter-country variance in the global prevalence of MSDs, which was greater in women compared to men and steadily rising in older age groups. The number of people with MSDs has increased globally as a result of a variety of major variables, including population expansion and an aging labour force [33]. Musculoskeletal disorders have been linked to an increase in disability, and this trend is expected to continue over the next decades. Although MSDs often do not pose a life-threatening hazard, they are frequently accompanied by discomfort, restricted mobility, and dexterity, which can result in early retirement from the workforce, decreased quality of life, and a decreased capacity to fully engage in society [34].

Multiple risk factors, including anthropometry, genetic history, age, sex, and a person's sexual orientation, play a role in the development of MSDs. The incidence of MSDs has been linked to a number of modifiable risk factors, particularly biomechanical overuse, organisational and environmental exposures, psychological risk factors, and other lifestyle disorders including smoking and obesity [35].

Psychosocial hazards have been more important in the research of factors that influence MSDs over time. However, the process is still being investigated, thus it is not yet feasible to link a single psychological risk factor to a particular MSD [36].

In middle Socio-demographic Index (SDI) areas and lower middle SDI regions, particularly in Asian nations, occupational hazards had the largest impact on disability-adjusted life-years (DALYs). The peak age at which MSDs first appeared changed from 35 to 39 years by 1990 to 50 to 54 years by 2019. Similar to this, the cost of DALYs peaked between the ages of 50 and 54 [37].

The issue of migrant labours, who are commonly known to work in "4-D jobs" (dirty, hazardous, tough, and discriminating), is another factor to take into account. The discriminatory element and other social factors of wellness that migrant workers encounter in their host nation while exposed to precarious labour are acknowledged by the addition of the fourth D, which has led to a high frequency of work-related MSDs (WRMSDs) [38].

We see a relatively high frequency of MSDs in low- and middle-income countries (LMIC), particularly in the agricultural, manufacturing, and service sectors. In Ethiopian working population, a recent systematic analysis of MSDs showed that the combined prevalence of work-related elbow discomfort, wrist/hand pain, knee/leg discomfort, foot/ankle pain, and hip/thigh discomfort in the preceding year was 19.7%. A sizable research from Pakistan that examined the incidence of MSDs among sawing machine users discovered that 200 participants, or 91% of them, exhibited signs of WMSDs in the previous year, with a substantial correlation between personal and occupational characteristics [37].

Each year, workplace-related deaths, illnesses, and injuries cost the US economy over $250 billion. Employers who adopt successful safety and health programmes saw a considerable increase in the output and profitability of their businesses [36].

The most prevalent rate was in the healthcare business, where the average number of missed workdays was just 8, compared to a median of 12 for MSD cases in the private sector. There were 77.1 MSD cases in the transportation and warehousing sector in 2018. The median number of days missed at work for MSD cases in both this industry and and the information industry was 26, and 33, respectively [35].

In 2016, there were 10,330 instances of back-related musculoskeletal disorders among nursing aides. Another 10,660 instances were reported among labourers and manual material movers. 15.6% of all back-related illnesses in 2016 came from these professions. By employment, different body areas are more frequently impacted by musculoskeletal problems. Over fifty percent of the cases experienced by nursing assistants in 2016 involved the back. Heavy tractor-trailer drivers reported a higher percentage of leg (16.3%) and shoulder (19.2%) injuries compared to other professions [35].

Despite a minor decline in MSD complaints over the past several years within the European Union, recent reports from the European Agency for Health and Safety at Work (EUOSHA) revealed that this health issue still affects more than half of the continent's workforce. The majority of these MSDs (45%) affect the back, 39% the upper body or neck, and 16% the lower body. From 65% in 2010 down to 50% in 2015, Italy's workforce percentage reporting any number of MSDs has dramatically declined [37].

Back pain was the most commonly reported health issue in 2018, followed by muscle pain during both the lower and upper limbs, making these illnesses the most prevalent ailment, accounting for 66.7% of all occupational diseases in Italy that were recognised in 2018. The two most common WRMSD types in Italy are dorsopathies and soft tissue disorders [36].

CRITICAL ISSUES IN EPIDEMIOLOGICAL STUDIES ON WORK-RELATED MUSCULOSKELETAL DISORDERS

The National Institute for Occupational Safety and Health, or NIOSH, published a paper in 1997 titled "Musculoskeletal Disorders as well as Workplace Factors. A Critical Assessment of Epidemiologic Evidence over Work Related Musculoskeletal Disorders Including the Neck, Upper Extremity, and Low Back," which is generally regarded as a "milestone." It concluded that a substantial body of reliable epidemiologic research revealed an ongoing connection between MSDs and certain physical factors, particularly physical strain [37].

The development of a wide consensus on case definitions has likely been delayed considerably by the frequent use of a broad vocabulary that encompasses disorders affecting many tissues and bodily areas in scientific literature and by international bodies. The term "MSDs" encompasses a wide range of illnesses; diagnostic nomenclatures and methodological methods have been developed within the area (multiple titles of the same disorder, nomenclatures that differ across various clinical specialties) [38].

When there are legal ramifications, like in the workplace, having a condition classified as a "disease" may have positive or bad effects on the workers, which may impact how they report symptoms. It's noteworthy that the International Labour Organisation (ILO) revised the guidance notes for the diseases included on the ILO List for Occupational Diseases in 2022, providing details and criteria to be taken into account in the identification and avoidance of such diseases. The recommendations are meant to be used by appropriate authorities, social security organisations, workers' compensation funds, occupational safety and health experts, medical professionals, employers, and employees, as well as those in charge of occupational disease notification, recording, prevention, and compensation programmes [40].

CURRENT TRENDS WITH EPIDEMIOLOGIC RESEARCH ON MUSCULOSKELETAL DISORDERS RELATED TO WORK

MSDs remain a common issue among employees everywhere. The tendency is supported by a recent EU-OSHA study. Despite laws and preventative actions, the prevalence of WRMSDs has risen between 54.2% in 2007 through 60.1% in 2013, throughout the EU's 28 member states. Age and gender, new formal employment relationships and work patterns, such as place of employment, working hours, or use of information and communication technologies (ICT), changing working practises, health behaviours and beliefs, psychosocial factors, and socioeconomic differences are all factors that influence the prevalence for MSDs in the workforce. Musculoskeletal issues may also be brought on by unhealthy lifestyles, inactivity, and growing obesity rates. Musculoskeletal problems and occupational sedentary exposure rise as the percentage of sedentary work increases [41].

There is currently a paucity of generally accepted diagnostic criteria, and the possibility of exposure misclassification is still up for discussion. Building consensus criteria for comparing the findings of various epidemiological research is the goal of a number of current efforts that attempt to increase estimates of the burden and natural history of MSDs as well as to comprehend the involvement of causative variables [40].

Van der Molen et al. carried out a scoping review to define diagnostic criteria for particular MSDs to be utilised in occupational healthcare programmes, surveillance, or research. Case definitions for WRMSDs and disorders that were published in peer-reviewed publications were compiled. Results showed a lack of standardization and documentation of the consensus criterion used for case definition in addition to a significant amount of variability in the definition of all MSDs, with the exception of low back diseases. Additionally, the authors advised that case definitions for WRMSDs incorporate exposure to work-related hazards for preventative reasons [42].

Sensors-based exposure assessment is another area that needs improvement. In the past few years, there has been an increase in interest in the use of wearable technology in ergonomics, particularly for the evaluation of physical aspects. For real-time movement monitoring and the evaluation of uncomfortable postures, single components and platforms that aggregate data from several devices are used; muscle activity or physical stress can also be collected [43].

Simultaneously, machine learning and artificial intelligence approaches have been developed to explore vast datasets in order to locate possible biomechanical, social, and psychological risk factors, monitor real-time WRMSD risk, and detect which employees may develop a WRMSD [44].

Prevalence

There can be differences in the epidemiology data for WMSDs between India and the rest of the world. Factors including uncomfortable postures and repetitive actions cause WMSDs, which impact millions of people worldwide. There are WMSD issues in several Indian sectors, including healthcare and manufacturing. Factors related to the workplace affect the prevalence rates. For example, globally, some continents have high rates of WMSD prevalence. For instance, WMSDs vary between 35.1% to 47% in America as well as 78.6% to 88% in Asia. The incidence of WMSDs in Africa varies as 44.1% to 94%. WMSDs are a prevalent source of morbidity that, among others, affects healthcare personnel worldwide. Different WMSDs have an influence on nurses, healthcare institutions, and the national economy. For instance, as seen in the USA of America, wherein musculoskeletal disorders account for an economic burden of between USD 45 and USD 54 billion annually, WMSDs cost significant yearly expenditures on nurses' medical treatment and compensation expenses [42-44]. In addition, at roughly 130 million healthcare contacts each year, WMSDs account for almost 70 million doctor office consultations. Musculoskeletal conditions are a serious public health issue that has an effect on how well nurses perform at work and have numerous negative personal, social, and financial effects. For instance, it has been stated that WMSDs have a negative influence on nurses' quality of job life, leading to more sick leave and absenteeism. In addition, Chang et al. revealed that nurses' quality of life is threatened by WMSDs. WMSDs are a significant workforce problem as a result, which makes premature retirement or absenteeism among nurses worse. It is important to identify the incidence of WMSDs and prioritise the solution in order to reduce overhead expenditures [44,45].

More efforts are required to expand the multifaceted interventions for WMSDs among nurses, according to Albanesi, Piredda, Bravi, Bressi, Gualandi et al. The most prevalent occupational hazards faced by nurses while performing nursing care duties in particular healthcare units are needlestick injuries, injuries to the body, stress and its effects on mental health, infections, chemical dangers, radiation exposure, as well as work-related exhaustion. These WMSDs have received the most attention from interventions so far. Amare et al. highlighted that WMSDs happen in a variety of medical settings, including units for people with intellectual disabilities [46].

Amare et al. highlighted that WMSDs happen in a variety of medical settings, including units for people with intellectual disabilities. A study addresses work-related musculoskeletal disorders (WMSDs) that nurses at a facility for people with intellectual disabilities encountered prior to the COVID-19 epidemic. Patients with recognised mental impairments that affect learning, problem-solving, and judgment are cared for in intellectual disability units. These impairments necessitate a variety of physical exercises. Intellectual impairment is characterized by a markedly diminished capacity for learning and using new abilities, as well as a diminished capacity for coping on one's own [45,46]. Meeting fundamental requirements (personal hygiene, dietary, and safety needs), changing positions, and providing intellectual assistance are some nursing services offered in an intellectually disabled unit. These tasks are completed in partnership using a multidisciplinary team. There is a significant risk of getting WMSDs within an intellectually disabled unit due to the necessary nursing care, but nothing is known about how often WMSDs are there [47]

In the healthcare industry, WMSD prevalence rates over a year range from 28% to 96%, including among nurses. Data from different sources throughout the world show that WMSDs are quite common in nurses. For instance, in Africa, Uganda found an 80.8% frequency of WMSDs among nurses due to the stress of lifting patients, carrying a large load, transferring patients from the floor to the bed, as well as working in uncomfortable positions [46]. According to Chiwaridzo, Makotore, Dambi, and Munambah's study, 82% of nurses employed in maternity, surgical, and medical facilities in Zimbabwe have WMSD. On the other hand, in Nigeria, it was discovered that at least 84.4% of the employed nurses had WMSDs during the course of their employment. According to research done in KwaZulu-Natal's healthcare institutions in South Africa, nurses are more likely to sustain injuries since part of their jobs requires them to manually move patients and bend, which is an important cause of WMSDs between nurses [48].

Numerous research have examined the incidence of WMSDs among nurses working in the healthcare industry as well as the contributing variables or root causes. These conditions can affect different body areas, such as the cervical spine, upper arm, wrist, and lower back, which is when back pain is most common. The most frequent WMSD among nurses is low back pain, which affects roughly 200,000 nurses annually and expenses the national healthcare system around GBP 45 million, or ZAR 87 391,395,000 billions of South Africa [46]. The majority of nursing care activities, such as patient care, washing patients, changing beds, taking care of wounds, and administering medications, are associated with these low back aches and other WMSDs.Given the nature of the work, nursing constitutes one of the professions in the healthcare industry where WMSDs are most common and challenging [45-47]. The common lifting of bulky items, moving patients, improper physical posture, fixed and constant neck posture, long-term, excessive shifts, psychological variables, job history, Body Mass Index (BMI), boosting working hours, and advancing age are some of the factors that put nurses at risk for developing musculoskeletal disorders. There is a need for more research in other units, such as the unit for people with intellectual disabilities, as these causes of WMSDs were reported among nurses employed in surgical units (17.8%), emergency departments (15.6%), outpatient departments (77%), and intensive care units (12.6%) [48,49].

Having the highest prevalence of diagnosed MSDs in the world, nursing is recognized as the occupation with the greatest risk of MSD development. The World Health Organisation (WHO) claims that as nurses' daily work schedules get busier, the problems associated with WRMSDs worsen. This is because of the physically taxing responsibilities performed in this career, which sometimes require uncomfortable postures when working with patients and considerable manual handling. Depending on the wards, hospital, and even the country in which they work, nurses may have different work-related musculoskeletal symptoms. These symptoms appear to be connected to several nurse occupational exposures to WRMSD dangers [50].

Although the lower limbs have recently drawn greater attention, the body parts with the highest prevalences of WRMSDs include the lower back, the neck, shoulders, the knees. They have forearms, hands, and ankles/feet. MSDs can affect the trunk, and upper, or lower extremities [51].

In a group of Asian nurses, studies have shown that the yearly incidence of musculoskeletal disorders (MSDs) is higher in at least one body part and/or region, ranging from 40 to 95%. In Western populations, the lower back, neck, and shoulders are the most severely affected body parts, with prevalences of 29–64%, 34-63%, and 17–75%, respectively [52]. However, a narrative analysis of the literature on MSDs during the year prior among female nurse staff demonstrated that the knee and ankle/foot areas were more commonly impacted. The incidence of MSDs varied between 7.2 and 77% in the knees and between 3.2 to 100% in the ankles. Between 8.5 and 10.5% of people had MSDs in their lower legs (the shins), while between 11 and 100% of people had them in their thighs and hips [53].

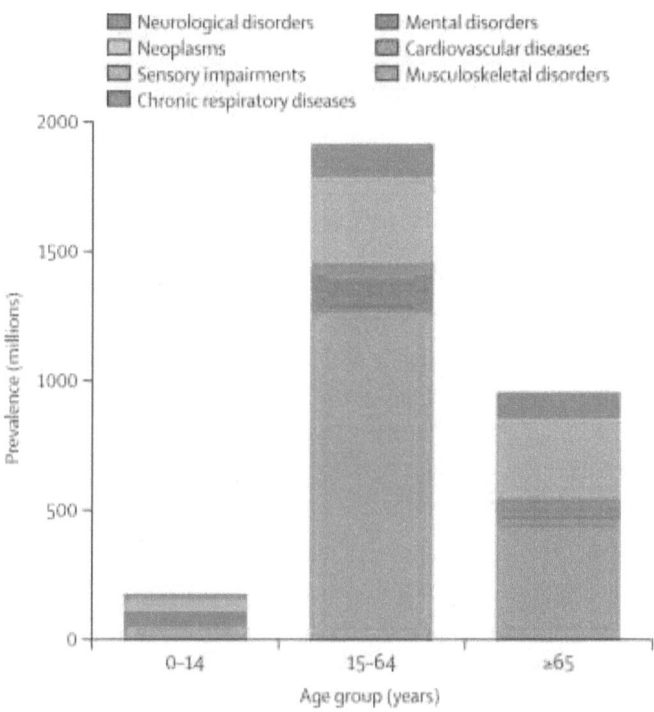

Figure 3: Categories of diseases where rehabilitation can be beneficial in 3 age groups (2019) [53]

Impact on Occupational Health and Productivity

Musculoskeletal diseases (MSDs) are pathological harm to the bones, ligaments, bones, muscles, nerves, and circulatory system that may impair the body's overall performance. Workplace-related MSDs (WMSDs) are musculoskeletal disorders (MSDs) that develop as a result of repeated activities such as bending, crawling, twisting, pulling, lifting, and tugging. The World Health Organisation has divided WMSDs into two groups: acute injuries and chronic injuries. Acute injuries are ones that have recently happened and might need to be treated right away by a medical practitioner. Chronic injuries develop gradually over time and result in enduring soreness and discomfort in the body; depending on the type and degree of the chronic injury and whether or not it affects performance at work, medical attention may also be necessary [54].

All MSDs and WMSDs have a considerable financial burden. In their safety index for 2018, Liberty Mutual Insurance (2018) stated that 13.7 billion dollars was spent throughout 2017 on overexertion injuries at work. According to the Bureau of Labour Statistics' 2018 report, there were over 2.9 million nonfatal workplace injuries in the private sector in 2016. Sprains, strains, and tears brought on by excessive activity were the most common type of injury, accounting for 30% of those incidents [55].

The natural next step to solve these issues is to concentrate on designating a healthcare expert who has experience in ergonomics, occupational safety, and the treatment of both MSDs and WMSDs. Physical therapists are uniquely positioned to assist with this spreading problem. Physical therapists can use education, ergonomics training, security at work changes, exercise prescription and monitoring, and hands-on manual treatments to avoid and treat musculoskeletal problems in the general population [56].

According to Pikaar (2012), ergonomics is the process of ensuring that employees are capable of carrying out their jobs safely in order to save expenses for businesses, boost workplace productivity, reduce WMSDs, and cut down on general absenteeism among employees. Employees who seek treatment and counseling on-site as opposed to off-site treatments spend much less on health care expenditures thanks to on-site physical therapy treatments, which include ergonomic education, training, and exercise [57,58].

References

1. Briggs AM, Woolf AD, Dreinhofer K, Homb N, Hoy DG, Kopansky-Giles D, et al. Reducing the global burden of musculoskeletal conditions. Bull World Health Organ. 2018;96(5):366–8.

2. Disease GBD, Injury I, Prevalence C. Global, regional, and national incidence, prevalence, and years lived with disability for 354 diseases and injuries for 195 countries and territories, 1990-2017: a systematic analysis for the global burden of Disease study 2017. Lancet. 2018;392(10159):1789–858.

3. Hagberg M, Violante FS, Bonfiglioli R, Descatha A, Gold J, Evanoff B, et al. Prevention of musculoskeletal disorders in workers: classification and health surveillance - statements of the Scientific Committee on Musculoskeletal Disorders of the International Commission on Occupational Health. BMC Musculoskelet Disord. 2012;13:109.

4. Sim J, Lacey RJ, Lewis M. The impact of workplace risk factors on the occurrence of neck and upper limb pain: a general population study. BMC Public Health. 2006;6:234.

5. Melhorn JM: Cumulative trauma disorders and repetitive strain injuries: the future. Clin Orthop 1998, 351:107–126.

6. Bureau of Labor Statistics: Nonfatal occupational illness data by category of illness. Washington, DC: US Department of Labor, 1995.

7. Tanaka S, Wild D, Seligman P, Halperin W, Behrens V, Putz-Anderson V: Prevalence and work-relatedness of self-reported carpal tunnel syndrome among U.S. workers: analysis of Occupational Health Supplement data of 1988 National Health Interview Survey. Am J Ind Med 1995, 27:451–470.

8. Yassi A: Repetitive strain injuries. Lancet 1997, 349:943–947.

9. Nainzudal N, Malantic-Lin A, Alvarez M, Loeser AC: Repetitive strain injury (cumulative trauma disorder): causes and treatment. Mt Sinai J Med, 66:192–196.

10. Yassi A, Sprout J, Tate R: Upper limb repetitive strain injuries in Manitoba. Am J Ind Med 1996, 30:461–472.

11. T.J. Armstrong, P.W. Buckle, L.J. Fine, M. Hagberg, B. Jonsson, G Kilbom, I. Kuorinka, B.A. Silverstein, G. Sjøgaard, E. Vu¨kariJuntura, A conceptual model for work-related neck and upperlimb musculoskeletal disorders, Scandinavian Journal of Work Environment and Health 19 (1993) 73–84.

12. T.J. Armstrong, L. Punnett, P. Ketner, Subjective worker assessments of hand tools used in automobile assembly, American Industrial Hygiene Association Journal 50 (12) (1989) 639–645.

13. L. Azaroff, C. Levenstein, D.H. Wegman, Occupational injury and illness surveillance: conceptual filters explain underreporting, American Journal of Public Health 92 (9) (2002) 1421–1429.

14. E.M. Badley, I. Rasooly, G.K. Webster, Relative importance of musculoskeletal disorders as a cause of chronic health problems, disability, and health care utilization: Findings from the 1990 Ontario Health Survey, The Journal of Rheumatology 21 (3) (1994) 505–514.

15. S.L. Baron, T.R. Hales, J. Hurrell, Evaluation of symptom surveys for occupational musculoskeletal disorders, American Journal of Industrial Medicine 29 (1996) 609–617.

16. B.P. Bernard (Ed.), Department of Health and Human Services, National Institute for Occupational Safety and Health, Cincinnati, OH, 1997.

17. Habib M, Yesmin S. A pilot study of prevalence and distributions of musculoskeletal symptoms (MSS) among paper based office workers in Bangladesh. Work. 2015; 50(3):371-378.

18. Silverstein B, Evanoff B. Musculoskeletal disorders. In: Levy BS, Wegman DH, Baron SL, et al., editors. Occupational and environmental health: recognizing and preventing disease and injury. New York (NY): Oxford University Press; 2011. p. 335-365.

19. Aptel M, Aublet-Cuvelier A, Cnockaert JC. Work-related musculoskeletal disorders of the upper limb. Joint Bone Spine. 2002; 69(6):546-555.

20. Holder NL, Clark HA, DiBlasio JM, et al. Cause, prevalence, and response to occupational musculoskeletal injuries reported by physical therapists and physical therapist assistants. Phys Ther. 1999; 79(7):642-652.

21. Crossley, K.M.; Stefanik, J.J.; Selfe, J.; Collins, N.J.; Davis, I.S.; Powers, C.M.; McConnell, J.; Vicenzino, B.; Bazett-Jones, D.M.; Esculier, J.-F.F.; et al. 2016 Patellofemoral pain consensus statement from the 4th International Patellofemoral Pain Research Retreat, Manchester. Part 1: Terminology, definitions, clinical examination, natural history, patellofemoral osteoarthritis and patient-reported outcome m. Br. J. Sports Med. 2016, 50, 839–843.

22. Hamilton, B.; Valle, X.; Rodas, G.; Til, L.; Grive, R.P.; Rincon, J.A.G.; Tol, J.L. Classification and grading of muscle injuries: A narrative review. Br. J. Sports Med. 2015, 49, 306.

23. Bahr, R.; Clarsen, B.; Derman, W.; Dvorak, J.; Emery, C.A.; Finch, C.F.; Hägglund, M.; Junge, A.; Kemp, S.; Khan, K.M.; et al. International Olympic Committee consensus

statement: Methods for recording and reporting of epidemiological data on injury and illness in sport 2020 (including STROBE Extension for Sport Injury and Illness Surveillance (STROBE-SIIS)). Br. J. Sports Med. 2020, 54, 372–389.

24. Valle, X.; Alentorn-Geli, E.; Tol, J.L.; Hamilton, B.; Garrett, W.E.; Pruna, R.; Til, L.; Gutierrez, J.A.; Alomar, X.; Balius, R.; et al. Muscle Injuries in Sports: A New Evidence-Informed and Expert Consensus-Based Classification with Clinical Application. Sports Med. 2017, 47, 1241–1253.

25. Chan, O.; Del Buono, A.; Best, T.M.; Maffulli, N. Acute muscle strain injuries: A proposed new classification system. Knee Surg. Sports Traumatol. Arthrosc. 2012, 20, 2356–2362.

26. Mueller-Wohlfahrt, H.W.; Haensel, L.; Mithoefer, K.; Ekstrand, J.; English, B.; McNally, S.; Orchard, J.; Van Dijk, N.; Kerkhoffs, G.M.; Schamasch, P.; et al. Terminology and classification of muscle injuries in sport: The Munich consensus statement. Br. J. Sports Med. 2013, 47, 342–350.

27. Pollock, N.; James, S.L.J.; Lee, J.C. British athletics muscle injury classification: A new grading system. Br. J. Sports Med. 2014, 48, 1347–1351.

28. Andersen JH, Kaergaard A, Mikkelsen S, et al. 2003a. Risk factors in the onset of neck/shoulder pain in a prospective study of workers in industrial and service companies. Occup Environ Med 60:649–654.

29. Andersen JH, Thomsen JF, Overgaard E, et al. 2003b. Computer use and carpal tunnel syndrome: A 1-year follow-up study. JAMA 289:2963– 2969.

30. Andersen JH, Haahr JP, Frost P. 2007. Risk factors for more severe regional musculoskeletal symptoms: A two-year

prospective study of a general working population. Arthritis Rheum 56:1355–1364.

31. Ariens GA, Bongers PM, Hoogendoorn WE, et al. 2001. High quantitative job demands and low coworker support as risk factors for neck pain: Results of a prospective cohort study. Spine 26:1896–1901; discussion 1902–1903.

32. Baker P, Reading I, Cooper C, et al. 2003. Knee disorders in the general population and their relation to occupation. Occup Environ Med 60: 794–797.

33. Bernard BP, Putz-Anderson V, Burt SE, et al. 1997. A critical review of epidemiologic evidence for work-related musculoskeltal disorders of the neck, upper-extremity, and low-back.

34. T.J. Armstrong, P.W. Buckle, L.J. Fine, M. Hagberg, B. Jonsson, G Kilbom, I. Kuorinka, B.A. Silverstein, G. Sjøgaard, E. Vu"kariJuntura, A conceptual model for work-related neck and upperlimb musculoskeletal disorders, Scandinavian Journal of Work Environment and Health 19 (1993) 73–84.

35. T.J. Armstrong, L. Punnett, P. Ketner, Subjective worker assessments of hand tools used in automobile assembly, American Industrial Hygiene Association Journal 50 (12) (1989) 639–645.

36. L. Azaroff, C. Levenstein, D.H. Wegman, Occupational injury and illness surveillance: conceptual filters explain underreporting, American Journal of Public Health 92 (9) (2002) 1421–1429.

37. E.M. Badley, I. Rasooly, G.K. Webster, Relative importance of musculoskeletal disorders as a cause of chronic health problems, disability, and health care utilization: Findings from the 1990 Ontario Health Survey, The Journal of Rheumatology 21 (3) (1994) 505–514.

38. Cieza A, Causey K, Kamenov K, et al. Global estimates of the need for rehabilitation based on the Global Burden of Disease study 2019: a systematic analysis for the Global Burden of Disease Study 2019. Lancet 2021; 396:2006–2017.

39. Safiri S, Kolahi AA, Cross M, et al. Prevalence, deaths, and disability-adjusted life years due to musculoskeletal disorders for 195 countries and territories 1990–2017. Arthritis Rheumatol 2021; 73:702–714.

40. WHO Fact Sheet ''Musculoskeletal Health'' Published 14 July 2022. Available at: https://www.who.int/news-room/fact-sheets/detail/musculoskeletalconditions. [Accessed 29 August 2022]

41. Steinmann S, Pfeifer CG, Brochhausen C, Docheva D. Spectrum of tendon pathologies: triggers, trails and end-state. Int J Mol Sci 2020; 21:844.

42. Challoumas D, Biddle M, Millar NL. Recent advances in tendinopathy. Fac Rev 2020; 9:16.

43. Macchi M, Spezia M, Elli S, et al. Obesity increases the risk of tendinopathy, tendon tear and rupture, and postoperative complications: a systematic review of clinical studies. Clin Orthop Relat Res 2020; 478:1839–1847.

44. Nichols AEC, Oh I, Loiselle AE. Effects of type II diabetes mellitus on tendon homeostasis and healing. J Orthop Res 2020; 38:13–22.

45. Odebiyi, D.O.; Okafor, U.A. Musculoskeletal Disorders, Workplace Ergonomics and Injury Prevention. In Ergonomics—New Insights; Intech Open: London, UK, 2023.

46. Yan, P.; Li, F.; Zhang, L.; Yang, Y.; Huang, A.; Wang, Y.; Yao, H. Prevalence of Work-Related Musculoskeletal Disorders in the Nurses Working in Hospitals of Xinjiang

Uygur Autonomous Region. Pain Res. Manag. **2017**, 2017, 5757108.

47. Attar, S.M. Frequency and risk factors of musculoskeletal pain in nurses at a tertiary centre in Jeddah, Saudi Arabia: A cross sectional study. BMC Res. Notes **2014**, 7, 61.

48. Arsalani, N.; Fallahi-Khoshknab, M.; Josephson, M.; Lagerström, M. Musculoskeletal Disorders and Working Conditions Among Iranian Nursing Personnel. Int. J. Occup. Saf. Ergon. **2014**, 20, 671–680.

49. Kasa, A.S.; Workineh, Y.; Ayalew, E.; Temesgen, W.A. Low back pain among nurses working in clinical settings of Africa: Systematic review and meta-analysis of 19 years of studies. BMC Musculoskelet. Disord. **2020**, 21, 310.

50. Franco, G. Commentary: Work-related Musculoskeletal Disorders: A Lesson from the Past. Epidemiology **2010**, 21, 577–579.

51. Nur Azma, B.A.; Rusli, B.N.; Oxley, J.A.; Quek, K.F. Work related musculoskeletal disorders in female nursing personnel: Prevalence and impact. Int. J. Collab. Res. Intern. Med. Public Health **2016**, 8, 294–298.

52. Mailutha, J. Prevalence of Musculoskeletal Disorders among Nurses in Kenya: Part 1, Anthropometric Data and MSDS. Int. J. Emerg. Technol. Adv. Eng. **2020**, 10, 158–163.

53. Cieza, Alarcos et al.. Global estimates of the need for rehabilitation based on the Global Burden of Disease study 2019: a systematic analysis for the Global Burden of Disease Study 2019; The Lancet, Volume 396, Issue 10267, 2006 - 2017.

54. Ahlstrom L, Hagberg M, Dellve L. Workplace rehabilitation and supportive conditions at work: a prospective study. J Occup Rehabil. 2013;23:248–260.

55. Bezner JR. Promoting health and wellness: implications for physical therapist practice. Phys Ther. 2015;95:1433–1444.

56. Bureau of Labor Statistics . Employer related workplace injuries and illnesses – 2016 [Internet] Washington, DC: U.S. Bureau of Labor Statistics; c2018. [cited 2017 Nov 9]. Available from: https://www.bls.gov/news.release/archives/osh_11092017.pdf.

57. Cecil R, Ross M. Effective worksite strategies and interventions to increase physical activity in sedentary workforce populations: the role of the physical therapists. Orthop Phys Ther Pract. 2017;29:56–62.

58. Chen X, Coombes BK, Sjøgaard G, Jun D, O'Leary S, Johnston V. Workplace-based interventions for neck pain in office workers: systematic review and meta-analysis. Phys Ther. 2018;98:40–62.

Chapter 2:

Ergonomics And Workplace Design

Ergonomics is the scientific study and practice of designing and arranging objects, environments, and systems to fit the capabilities and limitations of the human body. The primary goal of ergonomics is to optimize the interaction between people, their work, and their surroundings in order to enhance overall well-being, comfort, efficiency, and safety [1,2]. In simple words, it is the science of making a workspace or work desk as effective with respect to the anatomical structures of the human being as possible while lowering the risk of damage by balancing the demands of a job with the capabilities of the person and the work environment [1]. While in the past, minimizing the frequency of work-related musculoskeletal disorders (WMSDs) was considered the main objective of ergonomics, it also involves improving the effectiveness, quantity, quality, and comfort of the labour that is produced to maximize these elements while lowering worker injury, turnover, and fatigue/overexertion [1-3].

Successful ergonomics implementation can lower the risk of injuries and illnesses, boost worker productivity, and boost workplace happiness. If misused, it frequently can result in a rise in musculoskeletal disorders related to work (WMSDs). WMSDs are musculoskeletal disorders that develop due to working conditions or when an already existing musculoskeletal ailment gets worse due to those conditions or other workplace risk factors [1,2]. Jobs demanding frequent, forceful, or continuous use of the upper extremities, frequent lifting, pushing, or dragging of heavy things, or retaining uncomfortable positions for a lengthy period are a few examples of workplace risk factors [1,2]. The biggest ergonomics concern is frequently thought to be the lowering of WMSDs. Investigations show an association among certain specific movements and combinations of activities in the workplace (lifting, twisting, prolonged walking/standing, squatting, prolonged standing, and repetitive motions) placing people at a higher risk for developing WMSDs. Neck, back, and injuries to the upper extremities are some of the most frequent WMSDs [3]. Varicose veins, discomfort in the knees, hips, and ankles within the lower extremities, and postural imbalance/associated weakness; radiculopathy in the back, and spondylosis; Carpal Tunnel Syndrome, and De Quervain's tendonitis, and shoulder impingement disorders in the upper limbs are the most frequently cited symptoms of WMSD. The extent and type of WMSD vary greatly depending on the individual and method of injury [3,4].

It has been repeatedly shown that proper ergonomics application reduces WMSDs in a variety of workplace settings, lowering the number of ensuing missed workdays and wage losses as well as the risk of post-WMSD psychosocial problems. The application of ergonomics varies depending on the tasks being performed at the workplace and the person performing them. Females are frequently at higher risk for WMSDs than males due to their smaller stature, decreased physical strength output and instrument size/design being geared towards male stature [2,3].

Due to their influence on ergonomics as a whole and the possible consequences of WMSDs, psychological factors must also be taken into account when discussing ergonomics.

According to studies, psychosocial work elements such as workplace stress, work organization, and social support are associated with WMSDs. These elements may affect a person's ergonomic effectiveness and, thus, their possibility of WMSDs [4,5]. Links are additionally connected to the emergence of psychosocial illnesses, including depression and maladaptive pain responses, which, if treated improperly after WMSDs, may result in impairment. Another element that may have a detrimental effect on a person's receptivity to ergonomic education and increase their chance of acquiring WMSDs is fear of movement (FOM) [3-5].

CLINICAL SIGNIFICANCE

Working in repetitive, physically demanding, or ergonomic misaligned positions for extended periods of time increases the chance of acquiring WMSDs. Drivers, maintenance and construction workers, farmers, and healthcare professionals are some of the occupations where ergonomic misalignment is common. Surgeons, therapists, nurses, and dentists are the healthcare professionals most frequently associated with a higher risk for WMSDs, and each of these professions has particular ergonomic guidelines [5,6].

Professionals working in standing positions for prolonged time

The prolonged standing, uncomfortable postures, and repeated use of User Equipment devices that surgeons frequently use and raise their risk of postural strain and injuries due to repeated usage. The surgical crew can use the ergonomic modifications listed below to lower the chance of getting WMSDs.

1. Maintain your spine in a neutral position and keep your muscles relaxed. Every 10 or 15 minutes, take a quick pause to check your body's posture and make any necessary

modifications to ease any discomfort. To lessen the strain on joints, hold surgery instruments loosely, use different hands for simpler, repetitive activities, or squeeze the bottles uniformly with all of your fingers rather than just your thumb and index finger.

2. Position of the head and neck (as near to neutral as possible with a maximum of fifteen degrees of flexion advised; monitor with loupes and flashlights as the added weight tends to increase cervical flexion).

3. With a declination of 0 to 15 degrees, place the monitors 1 meter in front of the surgeon.

4. To ensure that the back is properly aligned, adjust the table's position to permit elbows at 90° to 120 degrees. In addition, to maximize ergonomic placement and alignment, alter and reposition the patient both before and during surgery.

5. It has been demonstrated that stretching exercises, including complete programs pre/post-op or intraoperative "micro-breaks," can minimize pain without lengthening the surgical procedure.

6. For individuals using the chair and foot pedals, make sure the chair has proper spinal support. Set up the foot pedals so that they are about a hip distance apart, at the same height, and with equal pressure on both feet. Ensure that the chair is at an appropriate height and that the knees are nearly or just barely bent at a 90-degree angle.

7. Use ocular extenders when using a microscope to avoid cocking your head forward. Take regular breaks from operating the microscope as well as focusing on a distant target when looking away from the microscope (every 10 to 15 minutes). When adjusting the microscope, use both hands to lessen the strain on the joints [6,7].

The above 7 points have been summarised in the figure below (Figure 4).

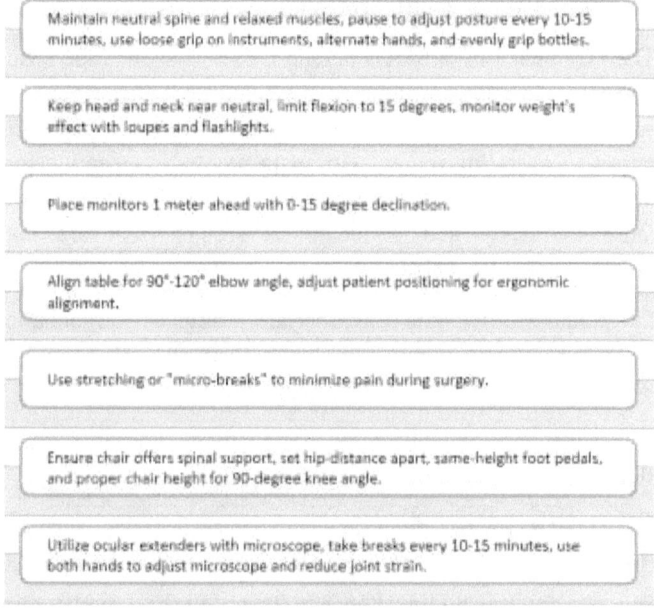

Figure 4: Points to remember for professionals working in standing positions for a long time

Laparoscopic techniques are used as a minimally invasive strategy to carry out routine procedures. Decreased postoperative recovery durations and postoperative rates of infection are advantages of laparoscopic surgery. However, comparable to an open technique, one of the main disadvantages of laparoscopic surgery is the surgeons' restricted field of vision and viewing angles. Laparoscopic operations can have negative ergonomic effects on surgeons when combined with extended static postures, which can cause the accumulation of lactic acid in the muscles and tendons. The ideal positioning of the trocar, table, monitors, and surgeon all have a significant impact on the ergonomics of laparoscopic surgeries [8].

Nurses and allied health professionals

The prevalence of WMSDs among nurses is significant, with nurses working in operating rooms having a higher rate. The same ergonomic risk factors that affect surgeons also affect nurses in operating rooms, with extra problems appearing for nurses who are caring for patients who must handle patients more frequently and frequently at weights that are not proportional to their size [7,8].

In addition to the appropriate surgical ergonomic recommendations, nurses can lower their risk of harm by putting these ergonomic strategies into practice:

1. Using anti-fatigue mats, supportive footwear, and stockings increases blood flow and minimizes edema.

2. Making use of appropriate transfer ergonomics, such as the use of lifting devices where necessary, the wearing of a gait belt, multi-team transfers, and the use of draw sheets, air-assisted transfer beds, or sliding boards. Positioning should be done before transfers are finished, which includes locking the brakes on the gurney, wheelchair, or bed, adapting bed height for ease of transfer, positioning the receiving transfer surface to the correct side of the patient, making sure the patient has the proper footwear (non-slip), and making sure the patient has received instruction so they can help with the transfer as much as possible [9].

Therapists

In addition to nurses, therapists frequently handle, position, and transport patients; therefore, the same ergonomic guidelines previously outlined for nurses also apply to their line of work. Physical therapists are also known to be at a higher risk for WMSDs because they do manual therapy on patients, which puts more strain on their upper extremities, especially their wrists and hands. Among the ergonomic recommendations to lessen these additional injuries are:

1. By having enough people, it is possible to distribute the workload and use support personnel as required.

2. To achieve the therapeutic benefit, the approach to treatment may be modified to include alternative therapies and the use of devices to minimize manual touch.

3. Ensuring that professionals have the resources they need to encourage their physical health is a preventative step [10].

Dentists

1. Ensuring that the instrument table and adjustable light are positioned correctly.

choosing tools with the best friction while requiring the least amount of force, such as those with suitable diameters, knurling or grooves, and curved shapes.

2. Using mechanized tools over manual ones to lessen the force placed on the hands and wrists.

3. Avoid using retractable or coiled hoses since they might cause your wrist and arm to tense up when they are stretched.

4. Position the patient horizontally.

5. Emphasis on maintaining proper seated posture, particularly when performing seated forward frequently bends enough to sustain lordotic curvature [11].

IMPORTANCE OF ERGONOMICS IN PREVENTING MSDs

Lesions in muscles, tendons, joints, ligaments, bones, nerves, and the blood circulation system are the hallmarks of musculoskeletal diseases (MSDs), likely to result in functional abnormalities. Musculoskeletal discomfort can strike at any age—infancy, adolescence, adulthood, or old—and last for a long time. Obesity, mental health issues, excessive sitting, strenuous activity, and smoking are the key risk factors in childhood and adolescence. sedentary behaviour, obesity, psychological discomfort, and a lengthy history of pain in adults. These elements play a role in the chronic pain linked to MSDs [12].

Regardless of the nature of the work activity, the prevalence of unfavourable health consequences has grown in groups who are occupationally active. Along with psychosocial issues, organisational behaviours, sociodemographic factors, and underlying pathologies, these situations may affect the development of WMSDs. One of the key issues in occupational health is WMSDs, which have substantial expenses, decreased productivity, and a lower quality of life in terms of health. Ergonomic interventions and workplace exercise are crucial to prevent injuries even though lowering workplace risk factors is challenging [13].

In fact, workplace exercise and ergonomic treatments enhance workplace quality, aid in the prevention or control of musculoskeletal problems, and give the adaptability and versatility required to complete jobs. The frequency of absences, medical leaves, exposure to risk factors, and potential injuries may be decreased using these types of measures. Since regular physical activity can help prevent or lower the risk of numerous diseases, workplace fitness programmes may also significantly improve employees' perspectives of their own work and quality of life and provide them with a stronger sense of well-being [14].

Prevention benefits employees, employers, and society at large. Identification, correction, and prevention of work-related diseases are essential in this situation because the workplace provides the necessary framework for proper assistance and attention to occupational health. Other issues to consider are low educational and professional qualification levels. WMSDs are directly influenced by occupation. For instance, repetitive and physically demanding tasks are a part of manual labor, traditional occupations like agriculture and fishing, or jobs with significant physical demands [12].

CLINICAL EVALUATION

A thorough medical history is necessary to get an accurate diagnosis. Diagnostic precision is also improved by physical examinations that include the probing of bone landmarks, posture analysis to look for abnormalities, and imaging testing. To increase performance, workplace risk, and occupational health analysis with an emphasis on the musculoskeletal system are essential [15].

A clinical evaluation of occupational ergonomics is a process of assessing the physical demands of a job and the individual's ability to perform those demands. The goal of the evaluation is to identify any potential risk factors for musculoskeletal disorders (MSDs) and to recommend ergonomic interventions to reduce those risks.

The evaluation typically includes a review of the worker's job description, a physical examination, and a range-of-motion assessment. The job description should be reviewed to identify the specific tasks that the worker performs, the tools and equipment that they use, and the work environment. The physical examination should assess the worker's overall health and fitness, as well as any specific risk factors for MSDs, such as muscle weakness or joint pain. The range-of-motion assessment should measure the worker's ability to move their joints through their full range of motion.

The results of the evaluation can be used to identify any potential risk factors for MSDs. These risk factors may include:

- Awkward or repetitive movements
- Heavy lifting
- Static postures (holding the body in the same position for a long period of time)
- Vibration
- Cold temperatures
- Poor lighting
- Lack of job control

Once the risk factors have been identified, ergonomic interventions can be recommended to reduce those risks. These interventions may include:

- Modifying the work environment, such as by providing better lighting or adjusting the height of the workstation
- Changing the way the job is done, such as by using different tools or equipment
- Providing training on how to perform the job in a safe and ergonomic way

The clinical evaluation of occupational ergonomics is an important part of preventing MSDs. By identifying and addressing the risk factors for MSDs, employers can help to protect their workers' health and safety.

Here are some additional methods that can be used in a clinical evaluation of occupational ergonomics:

- Questionnaires: Workers can be asked to complete questionnaires about their job duties, work environment, and any pain or discomfort they are experiencing.

- Observation: The worker's job performance can be observed to identify any potential risk factors.

- Videography: Video can be used to record the worker's job performance and to analyze it for ergonomic hazards.

- Biomechanical analysis: This involves using specialized equipment to measure the forces and stresses that are placed on the worker's body during their work activities.

The results of the clinical evaluation should be used to develop a plan of action to reduce the risk of MSDs. This plan may include ergonomic interventions, such as those listed above, as well as other strategies, such as providing workers with training on how to perform their jobs in a safe and ergonomic way.

By taking steps to prevent MSDs, employers can help to protect their workers' health and safety, reduce absenteeism and lost productivity, and improve morale.

Elaboration of Indian-Specific Scoring Systems and Scales for MS Disorders

Bathinda Musculoskeletal Index (BMI) (refer Table 7)

- Developed in Bathinda, India, specifically for the Indian population.

- Assesses disability and functional limitations arising from various MSK disorders, including arthritis, back pain, and limb disabilities.

- Uses a questionnaire covering activities of daily living (ADL) like bathing, dressing, eating, toileting, Bathinda Musculoskeletal Index (BMand mobility.

- Scores assigned to each activity based on difficulty level, with higher scores indicating greater disability.

- Useful for monitoring disease progression, evaluating treatment effectiveness, and prioritizing rehabilitation needs.

Table 7: Elaboration of Bathinda Musculoskeletal Index

Feature	Score	Description
Pain		
None	0	No pain
Mild	1	Painful on movement only
Moderate	2	Painful at rest and on movement
Severe	3	Constant pain, limiting daily activities
Morning Stiffness		
None	0	No stiffness in the morning
< 30 minutes	1	Stiffness for less than 30 minutes after waking
30-60 minutes	2	Stiffness for 30-60 minutes after waking
> 60 minutes	3	Stiffness for more than 60 minutes after waking

Range of Motion		
Normal	0	Full range of motion in all joints
Mild limitation (10-20 degrees)	1	Slight limitation in movement of some joints
Moderate limitation (20-50 degrees)	2	Moderate limitation in movement of some joints
Severe limitation (>50 degrees)	3	Significant limitation in movement of some joints
Functional Activities		
No difficulty	0	No difficulty performing daily activities
Mild difficulty	1	Slight difficulty performing some activities
Moderate difficulty	2	Moderate difficulty performing some activities, requiring assistance
Severe difficulty	3	Unable to perform many daily activities without assistance
ESR (Erythrocyte Sedimentation Rate)		
Normal (<20 mm/hr)	0	Normal ESR level
Mildly elevated (20-30 mm/hr)	1	Slightly elevated ESR level
Moderately elevated (30-50 mm/hr)	2	Moderately elevated ESR level

| Severely elevated (>50 mm/hr) | 3 | Significantly elevated ESR level |

Modified Lequesne Algometer (Table 8)

- · Adapted from the original Lequesne algometer, with 18 tender points specifically relevant to rheumatoid arthritis (RA) joint involvement.

- · Each point assessed with calibrated pressure applied by a spring-loaded plunger, measuring patient's pain response.

- · Tender point score calculated based on the number of points with pain and the applied pressure.

- · Widely used in India for diagnosing RA activity, monitoring disease progression, and assessing response to treatment.

Table 8: Scoring System for Modified Lequesne Algometer

Domain	Score Range	Description
	0-8	
	0	No pain
	1	Pain only after prolonged activity or unusual effort
	4	Pain on walking for more than 1 hour
Pain	8	Pain at rest or at night

	0-8	
Maximum Distance Walked	0	More than 1 kilometer
	4	Between 500 meters and 1 kilometer
	8	Less than 50 meters
Maximum Stairs Climbed	0-4	
	0	More than 10 steps
	4	Unable to climb 10 steps
Activities of Daily Living	0-4	
	0	Able to put on socks and tie shoelaces without any difficulty
	4	Unable to put on socks or tie shoelaces
Standing Up from a Chair	0-4	
	0	Able to stand up without using hands
	4	Unable to stand up without using hands
Total Score	0-24	

0	Normal
1-4	Mild
5-7	Moderate
8-10	Severe
11-13	Very Severe
14-24	Extremely severe

Western Ontario and McMaster Universities Osteoarthritis Index (WOMAC):

- · Originally developed in English, translated and validated in Hindi and other Indian languages.

- · Assesses pain, stiffness, and physical function in patients with osteoarthritis (OA) of various joints.

- · Three sub-scales: pain, stiffness, and physical function, each with questions specific to daily activities affected by OA.

- · Scores on each sub-scale and total score provide valuable information for diagnosis, monitoring disease progression, and evaluating treatment outcomes.

Component	Score Range	Description
Pain	0-20	
	0	No pain
	5	Mild pain
	10	Moderate pain
	15	Severe pain
	20	Worst imaginable pain
Stiffness	0-5	
	0	No stiffness
	1	Mild stiffness
	2	Moderate stiffness
	3	Severe stiffness
	4	Unable to move joint
Function	0-60	
	0	No difficulty
	10	Slight difficulty

	20	Moderate difficulty
	30	Severe difficulty
	40	Unable to perform activity
	50	Confined to bed
	60	Completely unable to perform any activity

Quick DASH (Disability of the Arm, Shoulder and Hand) (Table 9)

- · Originally developed in English, translated and validated in Hindi for the Indian population.

- · Assesses upper limb disability due to various MSK conditions in the shoulder, arm, and hand.

- · Short questionnaire with 30 items covering daily activities, pain, and general health.

- · Scores range from 0 (no disability) to 100 (severe disability), providing a clear picture of functional limitations.

- · Useful for evaluating treatment effectiveness, guiding rehabilitation planning, and monitoring progress in upper limb MSK disorders.

These scoring systems and scales offer valuable tools for healthcare professionals in India to:

- · Standardize the assessment of MSK disorders within the cultural context.

- · Enhance communication and understanding between patients and healthcare providers.
- · Monitor disease progression and treatment response accurately.
- · Prioritize and plan appropriate rehabilitation interventions.
- · Conduct research and compare outcomes effectively.

Table 9: Scoring System for Quick DASH

Score Range	Interpretation
0-10	No or minimal disability
11-20	Mild disability
21-30	Moderate disability
31-50	Significant disability
51-70	Severe disability
71-90	Very severe disability
91-100	Extremely severe disability, unable to perform most activities

WORKPLACE RISK ANALYSIS

Risk assessment can be done in a variety of methods at the moment, and the method used should be dependent on the evaluation's goals. Ergonomics are important in the examination of the workplace and in determining the level of risk to which employees are exposed while carrying out their duties [15,16]. The numerous approaches to research WMSD risk that we looked at included:

The REBA (Rapid Entire Body Assessment) Tool, a systematic method for evaluating full-body posture, was applied in research involving a variety of worker populations, including dentists, construction workers, meat cutters, employees at horse stables, rubber factories, and bicycle repair shops. These positions necessitate postures that increase the risk of MSDs, necessitating ergonomic analysis and functional research [11-13].

The risk was linked to continuous muscle contraction and repetitive movements in dentists75. The majority of the duties and postures performed by meat cutters and construction workers were reported to increase the risk of WMSDs. Bicycle repair shops urgently require ergonomic interventions to provide orientation on tools, workstations, and task use. The REBA approach offered predictors of MSDs in the neck, shoulders, elbows, upper back, lower back, hips, thighs, ankles, and feet for rubber factories. This technique further showed that the physical work required for maintaining horse stables represents serious ergonomic issues [13]. The effectiveness of therapies was also studied using the REBA approach. Ratzon et al. were able to prove that, after a brief follow-up time, nurses who participated in an ergonomic intervention programme had a reduction in their risk of developing WMSDs [11,12].

Yoon et al. were able to create a job rotation model to prevent WMSDs based on task groups of workstations with high and low workloads thanks to the quantification of risk provided by the REBA approach. To prevent injuries, this kind of approach might be recommended and modified for various occupational groups [13]. For use in Brazil, Lamaro et al. translated and culturally adjusted REBA. They do note that some reformulations are still required, though, and that biomechanical risk should be taken with caution [14].

OWAS (Ovako Working Posture Analysing System), or the OVAKO Working Posture Analysing System

OWAS is a heavy lifting evaluation tool. It evaluates the posture of the head, arms, legs, and back in relation to the required amount of force or weight. This scale has been used for several labour types [15].

According to OWAS, manual labourers were found to have a high prevalence of MSDs because of regular repetitive work that requires dangerous postures [16]. Brandl et al. analysed the most typical working positions in a semitrailer assembly facility and discovered that 26% of them can be detrimental to the musculoskeletal system. These authors assert that individual working posture-focused ergonomic therapies may result in better preventative effects than group-based strategies [15,16].

The use of OWAS enabled the demonstration of the increased risk of MSDs related to nearly all cooking job postures due to excessive repetitive motions. The same outcome was discovered for construction employees. OWAS in a vehicle assembly line revealed that corrective actions were required right away to stop the development of rotator cuff syndrome [15].

RULA, or Rapid Upper Limb Assessment

To determine the likelihood of causing injury to the upper limbs, RULA analyses posture and force. While this scale is one of the most commonly utilised to assess ergonomic risk across many occupational groups, more research is still required [16]. The whole worksheet has been demonstrated in Figure 5.

Compared to those without this ailment, computer office workers with musculoskeletal discomfort had higher RULA scores. When results are quantified in terms of RULA scores, ergonomic training may help lower the risk of MSDs in this population of employees [16].

Among dentists, a significant correlation between RULA scores and MSDs was discovered. The RULA score revealed that a submersible pump manufacturing facility's workstations displayed a high level of danger. The majority of body positions used by cooks were shown to be associated with a high risk of MSDs because of repetitive motions of the upper limbs. For pharmaceutical workers, a correlation between low back discomfort, RULA scores, and educational level was discovered [14,16].

The RULA scores indicated that there was an urgent need for ergonomic intervention in bicycle repair shops to offer technical advice on the use of tools, workstations, and task execution. This ergonomic intervention was aimed at assembly line workers at an electronic parts factory. Daneshmandi et al. discovered a decrease in the overburden to the neck and trunk after RULA was used [16].

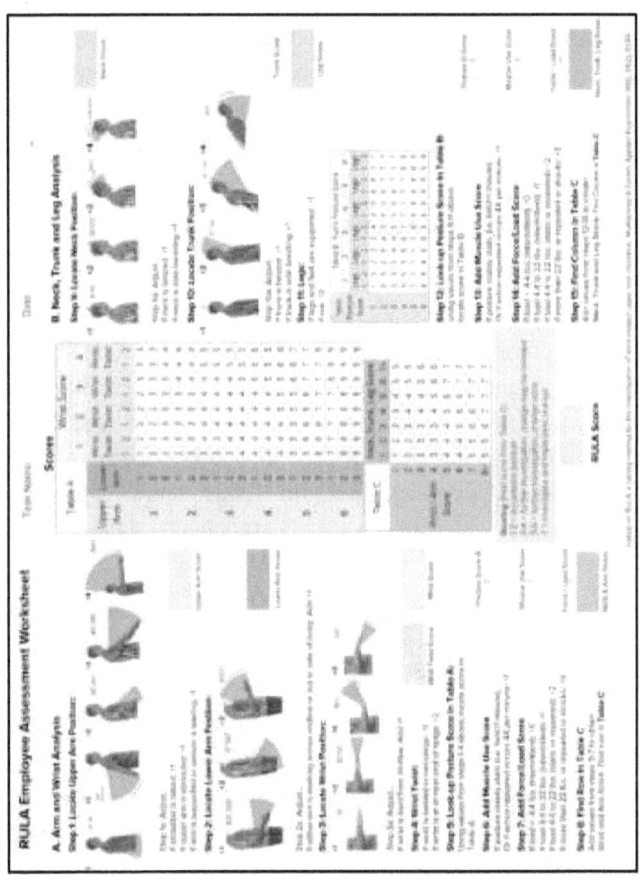

Figure 5: RULA Employee Assessment Worksheet

Index of Strain (SI)

The Strain Index (SI) was developed to evaluate posture and repetitive tasks involving the upper limbs, although little study has been done in this area. Among workers, lateral epicondylitis was correlated with SI scores [16, 17].

In order to reduce the risk of MSDs, SI enabled modifying tasks to be completed by employees who underwent a simulated drilling task. The SI risk group was found to be associated with a higher incidence of hand and arm symptoms in manufacturing workers. RSI, a freshly established improved version of SI, needs to have the adjustments it made reevaluated [17].

PRINCIPLES OF ERGONOMICS IN WORKPLACE

A standard on ergonomics principles relating to the design of work systems IS0 6385 (1981) Ergonomic principles in the design of work systems) was the first to be developed by IS0 TC 159 Ergonomics, documenting that this committee had adopted an ergonomics perspective that would lead to the development of the German DIN 33 400 (1975). As a result, this standard evolved into the fundamental ergonomics standard from which all subsequent ergonomics standards were formed [18].

In order to establish a broad frame of reference in which the other ergonomics standards might be incorporated and located, IS0 TC 159 decided to approach its standardization process from the top down [16,17]. It was immediately apparent that it would not be possible to create comprehensive ergonomics guidelines for every situation and that instead, more general criteria would be needed, which could be used to design consumer goods or work equipment for the specific issue at hand. This led to a policy that focused on fundamental standards that would be applicable to all types of equipment, products, and usage scenarios rather than product (specific) standardization. So, rather than, say, standards with anthropometric specifications for office chairs or automobile seats, the goal was to produce standards on fundamental anthropometric measures [15-18].

Designing work systems using ergonomics concepts (ISO 6385)

This fundamental criterion states that the design of work systems "shall satisfy human requirements," which can be thought of as a credo for applying ergonomics concepts to the creation of working environments. The application of ergonomics knowledge in the light of practical experience shall ensure the worker's health, safety, and productivity while at work, as well as contribute to more dependable, effective, and efficient system performance. With regard to the worker, IS0 6385 clearly goes beyond merely protective (avoiding negative effects) goals by ensuring optimal working conditions within a working system and thereby supporting worker promotion and task facilitation (in clause 4.3, for instance) [17,18]. Thus, it is made apparent by the standard that ergonomics considers system effectiveness and worker well-being from multiple angles, not just from a protective one. Contrary to the protective approach, it is interesting to notice that the social partners in the various nations do not all share the proactive perspective's acceptance [18,19]. In addition to outlining the goals of an ergonomic system design, IS0 6385 defines the fundamental vocabulary and ideas in ergonomics. The design of the workstation, work tools, work environment, and work process are then covered on a fairly generic level. For developing the work system in accordance with physical and psychological human qualities, basic principles and guidelines are presented. This contains specifications for the design that take into account biomechanical factors and anthropometric measurements, such as body measurements and movement principles. Additionally, some general guidelines are given for the layout, location, and design of displays and controls [19,20].

Again, at a fairly broad level, environmental factors like lighting, noise, and temperature are also covered, offering guidance for the design of work systems and leaving the specific information to specialized standards [16-18]. Although at a relatively basic level, some ergonomics rules for work organization are also discussed. Avoiding under and over-load is emphasized as a key aspect, and several recommendations are provided to help with this, including job rotation, job enlargement, job enrichment, and rest breaks [19,20].

As it stands, the revised version of this standard will place more focus on the idea of systems and the process of designing systems, including the assignment of tasks to humans or machines. Additionally, it will place more emphasis on task design and requirement principles, which were only lightly touched upon in the previous version of the standard but have since shown to be crucial and best addressed in the context of system design, particularly in the context of office work with VDTs [19,20]. Given that its assessment concepts are not sufficiently covered elsewhere, systems evaluation may eventually become a separate section of the standard on systems design. On the other hand, it appears to be quite necessary to offer some instructions on how to conduct an evaluation and/or how to show conformity with instructions, as described in ISO 6385 for system design, for instance. This is one of the issues with so-called "guideline standards" as opposed to "specification standards," where conformance can typically be checked with relative ease using (for instance) physical measurement processes [18-20].

Principles of ergonomics pertaining to mental burden (ISO 10 075)

The workload of the operator should be one of the criteria used to assess system design, or more generally the ergonomics design quality of any component, such as software design, as the workload has a direct bearing on both the debilitating effects of work on the operator and the development of the operator's capabilities and skills [17,18]. A separate standard (ISO 10 075) dealing with Ergonomic principles related to mental workload was developed within ISO because, as a result of increasing mechanization and automation, the mental workload is becoming more and more important and the area is typically not very familiar to the equipment or work system designer [18].

General Terms and Definitions

A terminology standard in the area of mental workload is thought to be necessary to ensure a better grasp of the terms, meanings, and concepts in this area. A specification in the area of mental workload appeared more than suitable, even though the broad idea of the stress-strain connection had already been established in ISO 6385 because the terminology was (and still is) employed in this field in wildly inconsistent ways [21]. This standard reserves the term "stress" for the stimulus side, despite the fact that the scientific literature contains notions that are stimulus-oriented, response-oriented, or interaction-oriented. The term "strain" refers to the organism's internal reaction, which can have either impairing or non-impairing effects. Warming up and learning are not impairments from mental workload, but "mental fatigue" and/or "fatigue-like states," such as "monotony" and "reduced vigilance," are. The standard does not address the long-term impacts of mental workload [19].

One of the most crucial things is the distinction between fatigue and fatigue-like effects, which can be determined by their recovery processes and antecedent situations (and thus require different design solutions to avoid them). Another interesting point is that the word "monotony" is only used to describe the internal response to a specific pattern of mental activity. Thus, "monotony" refers to the influence within the individual rather than the qualities of a work environment or task [19,20].

Design Principles

Guidelines for the design of work systems pertaining to mental burden are provided in Part 2 of ISO 10075. The ensuing mental workload of operators in a working system is acknowledged to be relevant, but selection and training are not addressed in the standard. The standard is organized in accordance with the definitions and ideas given in Part 1, providing information on how specific design features can affect mental workload and help prevent or reduce mental fatigue, monotony, satiation, and decreased vigilance [22]. It should be obvious that the standard's goal is optimization rather than minimizing mental workload (or stress), as required by European Directives. Avoiding underload is also crucial; avoiding overload is merely one of several factors. The key is to avoid any dysfunctional mental workload and to create an environment that encourages personal growth while also ensuring an optimal mental workload. The standard makes it obvious that there are qualitative differences in mental workload that must be taken into account in the design of work systems, rather than only the challenge of avoiding over- or underload on a unidimensional concept [20].

The presentation of information, the dimensionality, and dynamics of control movements, the development and use of mental models, the use of decision support systems, compatibility issues, and time constraints are some guidelines relating to the intensity of the mental workload with regard to mental fatigue. Guidelines for avoiding monotony address situations that are known to exacerbate it, such as repetition, a limited range of attentional demands, and monotonous ambient settings [18,19].

ASSESSING AND MODIFYING WORKSTATIONS FOR OPTIMAL ERGONOMICS

Assessment of ergonomics

Although the field of ergonomics has the necessary knowledge and skills for analysing occupational tasks and performance, there is little qualitative or quantitative data on the tools, equipment, and analysis methodologies utilised by practising ergonomists. Although the available evaluation tools have been listed, this information does not reveal how frequently or by how many ergonomists the tools are utilized [20]. Similar to this, there is limited evidence on these tools' usability, including factors that affect practitioners' choices on which tools to employ. Examples of qualities that most likely have an impact on use include time, necessary knowledge, and relevance. Ergonomists as a discipline have a stake in maximizing practitioners' performance because doing so can raise the value of goods and services for consumers [21].

Shorrock and Williams identified three crucial fundamental restrictions of ergonomics methodologies based on their own experiences: accessibility, usability, and contextual constraints. The term "accessibility" refers to the availability of publications, software, and intellectual property to practitioners. Tools' usability, for which there is little formal research, was defined as their usefulness and usability. The third restriction was contextual, which was concerned with the organizational traits and stakeholder impact within organizations where ergonomics is used [22,25].

This is multifaceted and comprises elements that eventually influence an organization's acceptance of a specific methodology and belief in the usefulness and relevance of the outcomes. Although these limits were not evaluated in the current survey, it is possible to deduce or at the very least speculate about how the results reflect the constraints [23,24].

The findings of a survey of the fundamental measuring tools, instrumentation-based direct measurement approaches, and structured observational-based assessment methodologies employed by U.S. Certified Professional Ergonomists (CPEs) were published in 2005 by Dempsey et al [26,27]. The Dempsey et al. (2005) publication has received numerous references as a source of knowledge regarding the application of evaluation techniques by ergonomics practitioners. Overall, the findings demonstrated that many U.S. CPEs utilized commonplace instruments like tape measures and digital cameras. The NIOSH Lifting equation and the Rapid Upper Limb Assessment (RULA) were two observational procedures that were fairly popular, but more sophisticated direct measurement techniques had far lower reported user rates [28,29].

Evaluation of ergonomics

Engineers rarely consider the viewpoint of the end user while creating a product or piece of work equipment by incorporating user feedback into the design process. Such a deficiency could affect the product/machine's quality and usability safety. Additionally, the employment of the workers is significantly impacted by their exposure to uncomfortable work situations, creating a serious societal issue [30].

A full approach to risk assessment is thought necessary to effectively address this issue, one that can integrate workplace and work equipment design with an investigation of working activities and workers' behavior while using it. In other words, an analysis of organizational, environmental, and job factors is required, focusing on those ergonomic features impacting the operator's behavior, such as human and individual characteristics, in order to achieve a safe interaction between the operator and the work equipment he or she is required to use on a daily basis [31].

There are several methods for assessing the physical requirements of workers. The Rapid Upper Limb Assessment (RULA) and Rapid Entire Body Assessment (REBA) procedures are the two that are most frequently used in this situation to assess the likelihood of work-related musculoskeletal disorders (WMSDs). While the REBA technique was discovered to be more sensitive to musculoskeletal concerns in the evaluation of postures in the health care and other service industries, the RULA approach is specifically intended to provide a rapid evaluation of the loads imposed by the postures of the neck, trunk, and upper limbs [30].

The Physical Demand Assessment (PDA) tool, for instance, is a procedure designed to gather information about the physical demands of a specific working task in particular body areas, based on the identification of ergonomic risks in the plant's production lines. Other approaches are those promoted by public bodies. For instance. While the use of such a tool necessitates a case-by-case analysis, it provides a framework of a general character for the qualitative evaluation of ergonomic risks. Engineers can do a job analysis of manual material handling exposures that entail lifting and lowering tasks using the "NIOSH equation". Such a tool has been employed as a reference manual for determining the recommended weight limit (RWL) for lifting tasks all over the world, particularly in its updated form that takes into account the examination of asymmetry and coupling elements [31]. This is frequently used in conjunction with the RULA and REBA tools to perform a thorough assessment of musculoskeletal disorders (MSDs) at work, but because it was created using anthropometric data from the North American population, an adaptation may be necessary if the anthropometric distributions of the sample under investigation differ [32].

Despite the widespread use of these techniques and the substantial body of research on the evaluation of working postures, some writers have noted the need for greater study into the creation of more useable strategies. De Galvez et al. specifically emphasized the requirement for practical assessment tools to make it easier to incorporate ergonomics concerns into occupational risk assessment processes. Li et al. also noted that little study has been done on the assessment of physical demands and working conditions in the industrial sector, where operators' uncomfortable body position is one of the most important ergonomic risk factors [32]. As a result, they encouraged the use of more extensive methods that could record all the data required for risk assessment (such as the task's duration). Musculoskeletal diseases, which are frequently accompanied by pain and exhaustion, might, in fact, be brought on by an improper working posture. Such a scenario can even affect how employees are positioned, which can result in mistakes that raise the likelihood of dangerous circumstances and lower the quality of work output [33].

The ISO 11226 standard (which was reviewed and approved in 2018) suggests a two-stage process for evaluating workers' static postures, taking into account five different postures relating to the trunk, head, shoulder, forearm/hand, and legs. The standard includes technical details on how to conduct the acceptability evaluation for each of these components. The fact that this information is disjointed and that the bulk of the suggested criteria can be difficult for non-expert evaluators to understand limits the application of this information in real scenarios [34].

Computer workstation ergonomics

The prevalence of computers in the workplace is rising everywhere. The percentage of American households having a desktop or laptop computer increased from 9% to 79% between 1984 and 2015, demonstrating the growth in home computer use for business and education over the past few decades. Only 10% of US workers worked from home (WFH) prior to the COVID-19 epidemic, according to estimates. Until the implementation of social distancing caused a sudden and sustained increase in the number of employees WFH since March 2019, WFH was a coveted benefit discouraged by most employers due to cybersecurity concerns, the cost of setting up a home office, and the belief that optimal job performance required physical presence [35].

Some musculoskeletal (MSK) pain and symptoms have been linked to worker and work method interactions with outdated, broken, unadjustable, or ill-fitting equipment in both domestic and professional contexts. Multiple factors, including physical and biomechanical expositions, work expectations and organization, workstation designs, inadequate postural support, and personal and job-specific psychosocial concerns, all contribute to the developing MSK symptoms [36]. Awkward, persistent, non-neutral postures and repeated motions that may heighten muscle tension in the upper limbs are physical risk factors associated with computer workstations that may be related to MSK symptoms. Szeto et al. used photographs of the workstation and a questionnaire regarding computer use and MSK symptoms to evaluate the computer workstations that primary school students in Hong Kong used at home. They came to the conclusion that using the wrong equipment could cause children to adopt poor posture [37].

Patients regularly seek therapists for recommendations on computer workstation designs. Additionally, they could be asked to offer business advice on workstation configuration, dangers, and suggestions in private or corporate settings. In the first instance, a patient is being treated by a doctor. In the second scenario, the client may not necessarily be the employee seeking specialized examination and treatment for MSK problems but rather the employer or employee requesting evaluation of the workstation and workplace difficulties. In this instance, the clinician is addressing particular client needs [38].

Clinicians frequently rely on client self-evaluations and descriptions of computer workstations as the primary sources of objective data about workstation setup, postures, and completed tasks. For instance, the Rapid Office Strain Assessment (ROSA), a reliable and effective tool created for use by trained professionals to assess computer workstations in an office setting, is based on extensive research on computer and office work as well as the Canada National Standards for Office Ergonomics. The validity of employee self-assessment in relation to expert assessment of risk exposure levels was studied by the authors, who discovered considerable discrepancies between worker ROSA ratings and those of trained observers, notably in relation to mouse and keyboard exposure and postures [39].

There are many simple computer workstation checklists that can be utilized to methodically improve remote photographic assessment. Due to the wide variance in stature, race, gender, anthropometric dimensions, and small variations across international standards, checklists are often predicated on the idea that no single evaluation applies to all circumstances and body types [36]. Despite these discrepancies, a trustworthy and tried checklist, like those recommended in this review, facilitates a more thorough discussion about all aspects of the workstation, such as setup, general posture, chair issues, keyboard and mouse position and types, monitor and phone positions, the impact of glasses on viewing, placement of documents, footrests, and lighting, improving understanding of component-worker interactions as well as the impact of equipment. Recent checklists offer some considerations relevant to sit-stand concerns, and the office ergonomic parts of OSHA and CAL OSHA have checklists tailored specifically to offices [38].

All of these materials offer thorough details on office workstation components, justifications for evaluation and use, and helpful graphics that can enable an evaluator and client to have a productive conversation [39].

The therapist must comprehend the ideal computer workstation postures and link symptoms or issues of concern to the interaction of the work components in order to move from collecting and receiving data to addressing the work setup and methods, interpreting information, and ultimately determining suggestions for equipment and postural improvement [35]. The various parts of a computer workstation and where they are placed may need to be taken into account. In order to enable and attain a neutral posture for the neck, shoulders, elbows, wrists, and back, which is collectively described as an upright sitting posture on a chair with elbows, hips, knees, and ankles positioned at around 90° angles, the evaluation and discussion should focus on these areas. According to Woo, White, and Lai, good sitting posture is essential for maintaining back support and reducing low back discomfort. They recommended that feet be on the floor, as recommended by OSHA 21, or supported by a suitable footrest. In general, the upper arms should be near the body and not outward or to the sides. The elbows should be flexed 70 to 90 degrees, the wrists should be neutral, and the head and neck should be straight ahead [36].

Chair

Van Niekert, Louw, and Hillier recommended starting with the workstation's chair, which is the most easily adjustable and possibly influential piece, in order to achieve perfect posture when using a computer. The chair positions the client so that they can use the keyboard, mouse, and monitor. It also serves as a foundation of support for their legs, back, and head. Although generally speaking, Van Niekert found limited evidence that a proper chair was directly associated with decreased severity, intensity, and duration of the MSK symptoms associated with prolonged sitting, Rodrigues, Leite, and Lelis found that poor chair fit or adjustment led to increased ROSA scores and user discomfort [37].

The right chair height is crucial. The popliteal space may experience more pressure if the chair is too high, while the low back and ischial tuberosity may experience pressure if the chair is too low. The lateral sitting shot will demonstrate whether the goal postures of knees slightly below hip level with feet supported and hips flexed at about 90 degrees will be visible. This image can be enhanced by the chair height measurement: shorter workers often require a seat height of 17" to 19", while taller clients may want a seat height closer to 20". With feet on the floor and a seat height of 20", it is likely that a shorter client's hips and knees won't be at 90 degrees, so the seat height should be lowered or foot support should be offered as necessary [37].

The depth of the seat pan is essential for supporting the back while seated. MSK symptoms may develop if a chair used at home or at a workplace does not fit a client properly, particularly if it is non-adjustable, too large, too tiny, or if the client is unable to change these chair components. If the seat pan is too short, pressure on the posterior thigh may lead to lower back muscular pain, while a seat pan that is too lengthy may force customers to sit forward without any support for their lower and middle backs. When a client is seated all the way back in the chair, a proper seat pan depth often leaves 2" to 4" of space between the front of the seat and the client's posterior knee [37].

In many ergonomic chairs, the seat pan angle can also be changed, however, customers are frequently unaware that the seat may be "pitched" downward and may not know how to change this. In most circumstances, a downward pitch is not desirable since it might increase trunk muscular activity and lead to sitting-related weariness. If the perch position is required, a modest downward pitch may be employed, although a forward pitch of around 15° is typically recommended. The client is positioned forward on the chair in this declining or perched position, which can be utilized sometimes to sit in a different posture [37].

Armrests

The use of armrests is debatable. According to some writers, using armrests may lessen the strain on the muscles in the neck, shoulders, and arms. However, if the armrests are excessively high or wide, clients may have to lift their shoulders or abduct them in order to go about. The authors recommend that armrests be easily movable, if not removed, to allow for the arms to be in a neutral posture when using the keyboard and mouse. Measurements or photographs can assist in identifying whether shoulders are elevated or armrests are excessively high, signaling the need to have a conversation about lowering or removing the armrests [38].

Desk

The desk's height (sitting and standing, if both are utilized), available workspace, and organizational capabilities should all be considered. The recommended height for keyboard desks is between 22" and 28", depending on the client's sitting height, and 37.4" to 45.5" when the client is standing. The height is calculated by the distance from the floor to the elbow or hand when the client is seated or standing in the proper posture. This position reduces stress at the elbow and wrist while allowing the shoulder to relax. Most women and many men will find the traditional fixed desk's height of 28.5" to 30" to be excessively high for using a keyboard and mouse. According to Woo, if a desk is just 5 to 10 cm (2 in. to 3 in.) above the floor to elbow height with the shoulders relaxed, the client will frequently lift the shoulders to use the keyboard, which will cause them to become tired and experience pain in the thoracic and cervical region [38].

Keyboard and Mouse

If a workstation is too high for using a keyboard and mouse, offering a completely adjustable keyboard tray that can be flat (not slanted upwards) or positioned with a slight negative incline is a useful solution, especially if the client has wrist or elbow issues. When typing for extended periods of time, Rempel, Keir, and Bach recommended avoiding wrist extensions more than 30 degrees, whereas Woo advised keeping wrist extensions at or below 15 degrees to reduce wrist strain and advocated using a keyboard tray if practical. To prevent shoulder elevation, which could happen if you reach for the mouse above keyboard height, or wrist extension, which could happen if the mouse is lower on a flip or slide-out extension, the keyboard tray should have enough room so that the keyboard and the mouse are at the same height [39].

Typically, a space 26" to 30" wide is needed for this, or an area under the desktop big enough for a full-sized keyboard tray. The tray shouldn't have any "under tray" components that could hit the client's thighs, and it should be able to independently adjust for height, angle, and/or tilt [37].

The client's chair may be raised to provide a more comfortable posture for the elbow and wrist if a keyboard tray is not available or able to be mounted to the work area. In this case, a footrest is needed to support the back and legs. By replicating the 90° flexed hip and knee posture, situating the ankle as if it were on the floor, and measuring the distance from the volar surface of the foot to the floor, the appropriate footrest height can be estimated. The primary author of this review has noticed that it is more difficult for the client to enter and exit the workstation by putting their feet on the floor when they are sitting too high and utilizing a footrest [39].

According to NIOSH, the type of keyboard used will depend on the duties being performed as well as the operator's skill. On the internet, you can find a variety of split, adjustable, and curved keyboards that you can discuss with your client. There is scant evidence that any one type is best for all applications and users, despite the fact that most are made to moderate forearm pronation or wrist deviation. Additionally, prolonged laptop keyboard use has been linked to an increase in non-neutral neck, shoulder, elbow, and wrist postures as compared to using a full-sized keyboard [39]. Many mouse devices, such as normal, vertical, trackball, or roller forms, are surprisingly varied in their usage styles and designs. The type and positioning of the mouse are considerably more important now that mouse usage surpassed keyboard usage in 2008 and probably continues to do so today [40].

A non-standard mouse design should be supported by solid clinical evidence relating to MSK symptoms. For instance, a vertical mouse may not reduce wrist motion and extensor muscle strain that may be associated with lateral epicondyle symptoms, nor would a trackball mouse lessen right thumb discomfort brought on by gripping the mouse incorrectly or by hand size. To reduce the frequency of gripping and wrist movements in these situations, it could be wiser to suggest that the client learn to operate the mouse on the opposite side. By altering the clicker button and advising moderate use to develop competence and tolerance, this can be accomplished more readily [39].

Monitor and phone

Incorrect monitor positioning can directly affect eye fatigue as well as neck, back, and lumbar discomfort. If too high or too low, neck flexion or extension may happen, which causes muscle fatigue in the stabilizers of the neck and shoulder. This is especially true if the customer is wearing bifocal or progressive lenses, or if they are trying to see between a computer screen and desk-bound documents. When using dual monitors, if the monitors are not centered with the keyboard and user trunk, if hard copy papers are on clips or stand next to the monitor, or if the monitors are not centered, neck rotation is connected with higher cervical and thoracic discomfort [40]. By modifying the height and placement of monitors to correspond with the most frequent use and taking into consideration the position and style of copyholders, non-neutral neck postures should be minimized over time. When viewing a display that is too far away or has a very small print, the trunk may flex, resulting in cervical extension and eye strain. Screens should, on average, be 63 to 85 cm (24" to 33") away from the client, according to the authors [41].

Workstation organization

Office work is regarded as sedentary, but according to Springer and Woo, using a computer while seated is dynamic because users frequently adjust their posture in their chairs, and if tasks are varied, they use equipment in a variety of sequences, positions, and intensities to complete various tasks at the same station. According to Emerson and Finch, alterations to one component or work element may have an impact on the positioning of other components and the posture of the worker because of the interaction between the user and the equipment. The organization of the tools used can benefit from an understanding of near, midrange, and far reach in relation to the performance of work tasks [41].

Sit-stand workstations

Interest in sit stand desks has grown as more studies about the harmful impact of extended sitting on general health have been widely accepted. Inactive work postures and a sedentary lifestyle have been linked to heart disease, type 2 diabetes, low back pain, and other MSK symptoms, according to research. During the workday, many customers should aim to change their posture, include movement away from the desk, and alternate often between sitting and standing. Although studies agree that we should "sit less and move more," authors emphasize that there is no single ideal rate of movement [39]. According to Karol51, standing for several periods of 30 minutes or less throughout the day could reduce the detrimental effects of prolonged sitting. Numerous types of research emphasized the significance of informing clients about the advantages of sit-stand as well as the significance of social and motivational support, including prompts, group reinforcement, and cell phone reminders, in order to produce long-lasting changes in sit-stand behavior. Better compliance was linked to the usage of electric height-adjustable workstations as opposed to mechanical ones and instruction on appropriate equipment heights and uses. Whether to sit or stand while working may also depend on the task at hand because activities requiring fine motor skills, such as writing, manipulating paper, and data analysis, were best carried out while seated [40].

The ideal arrangement for standing has been said to resemble sitting posture in terms of the shoulder, elbow, and wrist. However, Lin et al. discovered that individuals in a research of 20 people preferred the display to be 6 cm higher and the keyboard, mouse, and and monitor to be closer to the desk edge when they were standing as opposed to when they were seated. They also highlighted that a lower desk height in relation to elbow height could promote wrist extension. Sit-stand workstation alternatives might be overwhelming, so it's important to carefully consider user function and fit in relation to any MSK symptoms. Electric height-adjustable equipment may be the most effective for a client with back or upper-quarter limitations or MSK symptoms to ensure that the patient moves between sitting and standing position without utilising mis-aligned or forceful postures that demand a forceful grasp to elevate or lower the equipment [41].

The home workstation

If the employer hesitated to approve the cost of equipment duplication, the client may have carried equipment from the corporate office home with authorization, or the client's home workstation may contain equipment that is comparable to that in the corporate office. The home workstation can still bring particular difficulties, though. Employees might not have the necessary storage space or transportation options for the many pieces of corporate office equipment. They might therefore employ tools that do not encourage good postures. Employees might lack the necessary components, and if financial assistance is not offered, they might be reluctant to pay the component costs. Employers who are aware of potential issues with home workstations have offered online recommendations for ergonomic home office components, as well as stretches and other support services (examples include Chubb 2020, Liberty Mutual 2020, and Travellers 2020). To establish better at-home working postures and to give the clinician a starting point for a conversation with the employer regarding necessary equipment, clients should be encouraged to go over these documents with the therapist [42].

Employers frequently permit employees to use computers outside of the office. Despite being suitable for brief, occasional usage, Yu et al. found that when laptops are used full-time and daily, there are noticeable posture changes of the neck, elbow, and wrist, as well as more shoulder elevation than with desktop computer use. If a laptop serves as the primary computer, an additional keyboard, mouse, and display should be available, or at the very least, an external keyboard and mouse can be utilized while the laptop is positioned at a more comfortable height on a desk or table, allowing the shoulders to relax [40].

The therapist's role

There is no "magic bullet" that ensures MSK discomfort is avoided. Darragh, Harrison, and Kenny discovered that participatory ergonomics and training were useful in ensuring client involvement with the recommendations and long-lasting behavioral changes that will sustain improved work-related health. Better carryover and adaptive change were observed in microscope workers sitting in postures similar to computer workers when personnel was involved in equipment decisions, reinforced good posture, and used equipment [41].

The therapist acting as a consultant in an ergonomic consultation practice concentrates on responding to the employer's referral question, which in the case of the article is "Does the computer workstation need to be modified?" The therapist-consultant may have a suspicion that the client requires an upper limb therapy evaluation to address movement dysfunction that may be a contributing factor to the client's reported MSK pain and symptoms, but in this case, it is typically not the consultant's responsibility to provide an evaluation or therapy. Outside of the specific consultative position, this can be offered for consideration [40]. In contrast, a therapist who assesses and treats a client's upper limb MSK pain in a conventional outpatient clinic setting is unable to create a comprehensive plan of care without first conducting a computer workstation evaluation. The outpatient clinic's demands on productivity, patient coverage, and monitoring may prevent therapists from conducting on-site, in-person workstation evaluations. The therapist has a consistent technique of data collection and evaluation with the remote and/or virtual approach presented in this study. This method enables the therapist to prescribe the right workstation improvements and patient education to help resolve MSK discomfort and symptoms [42].

ERGONOMICS TOOLS AND EQUIPMENT FOR DIFFERENT OCCUPATIONS

Recently, producers, consumers, and researchers have all expressed a renewed interest in ergonomic hand tool design. The tool had to meet the needs of the maximum number of users feasible, do the purpose for which it had been built satisfactorily, and be as affordable as possible. As a result, a particular tool was created to be used by all possible users. Recent years, however, have seen a shift in thinking, and tool design now incorporates new ideas of greater comfort and decreased biomechanical solicitation with respect to users' functional capacities. There are numerous factors influencing this growth. The most significant trend is the increase of work-related musculoskeletal diseases of the upper limbs (WRMSD), which are especially prevalent in businesses that use hand tools [43]. According to a study (Myers and Trent, 1988), WRMSD was responsible for 24% of all reported hand tool injuries. Second, new types of production process organization (just in time, ISO 9000 quality certification), as well as the development of new technology (artificial intelligence, robotics), have all had an effect. These elements call for employees to be more involved in the work process itself and to have a wider variety of skills and knowledge [44]. From this background, new tool requirements have been developed. Last but not least, the competition amongst hand tool manufacturers has expanded the range of expertise needed by manufacturers, including ergonomics, in order for them to react to market forces. In reality, when making hand tools, tool manufacturers must consider three new categories of needs. These include understanding the various ergonomic stages involved in the design process, including ergonomics into the design process, and designing hand tools with a variety of considerations in mind [43].

Ergonomics integration into the design process

The design process should be properly organised. In fact, it is now commonly acknowledged that the initial stages of the design process determine 75% of the overall costs associated with the development and industrialisation of a product [44].

Method in a design process refers to a strategy in which various "models" (language, technical experience, know-how, etc.) are brought together with various "tools," on the one hand. Here, "tools" refers to all the methods used to examine how a component or entire design process functions [44].

A general design approach includes several project phases (definition of needs, specifications, general and detailed design), as well as a group of project participants (marketing, design, production). If the project is to be successful, the chosen strategy must achieve the highest level of integration of these many components [45].

The project participants and phases were envisioned using traditional design process methodologies in a sequential order. Such an approach has the effect of making it very difficult to incorporate ergonomics into the design process. Two strategies are suggested for overcoming these challenges. On the other hand, spiral models for phase organisation should be employed, which are iterative models. On the other hand, it is advisable to use concurrent engineering to control the many process protagonists [44].

The various ergonomic stages in the design process

There has been a re-evaluation of the purpose and meaning of the design process as a result of growing knowledge that (a) the user, (b) the tool, (c) the workplace, (d) the environment, and (e) the task itself are inextricably intertwined [43,45]..

The three factors that were just highlighted do, in fact, all interact with the other two. Only through utilising ergonomics can this goal be accomplished. There are basically three stages:

• **Stage 1:** After careful observation of the work process and work environment, definition of user requirements and expectations. During this phase, employee qualities (training, anthropometric measures, etc.) are also determined. The examination of user requirements and work processes leads to the development of tool specifications.

• **Stage 2:** Based on tool specifications and laboratory simulation, a new tool prototype is designed, and its biomechanical solicitation is compared to that of the tool that was previously in use. All other phases pertaining to tool function, styling, and other aspects are included in this stage, including concept modelling, functionality modelling, and functional prototypes.

- **Stage 3:** Prototypes are tested by a large sample of users in actual professional settings after the formal conclusion of stage 2. The trial should last a considerable amount of time (a few weeks), and input on how users feel about the new tool should be routinely sought after using a method similar to that employed in the first phase. The tool can be regarded as properly certified for the situations in which it has been tried and tested if good results are attained. Before making a final decision, users must be instructed and motivated to use the prototypes for a considerable amount of time [45,46].

The criteria used in hand tool design

Tool Design

The main factors to consider when it comes to tool design are tool weight, centre of gravity, handle form and dimensions, handle length, handle material and texture, trigger, guards, inclination of the tool, handle relation to the functional part of the tool, vibration, and reaction torque [46].

User Elements:

The design of hand tools is greatly influenced by anthropometric factors such as age and gender, right- and left-handed users, experience and technique, training, and so on [46].

Workstations, tasks, and environmental factors:

Workplace considerations include the proper tool for the job, posture, the surrounding environment, the usage of gloves, the tool supports and reaction torque bars, and tool maintenance [46].

Agro-based workers

Since the commencement of ergonomics operations in India, the application of ergonomics in traditional village technology, work tools, and work methods that go along with the existing abilities and know-how knowledge has continued to be the component of the highest emphasis. Low levels of productivity are the result of equipment design flaws that unintentionally ignore ergonomic considerations. With the reference parameters to evaluate the design development process for enhancing productivity and their general wellbeing, the efficient design application in agro-based engagement is praiseworthy [47].

Status of the job and tool development

Assam's industries that produce tea leaves, pineapple as a fruit, and pickles (from other locally accessible raw materials) rely heavily on female work. Both industries require a variety of arm and finger movements, and how they are used depends on the workers' experience, skill level, and level of weariness. It was crucial to consider the necessity for any work tool creation in order to boost productivity. Women often work on tables while standing or sitting on the floor, using regular stools as seating devices. Only manual labour is required to peel, remove the eye, and core the pineapple's hard centre [48]. The short pineapple harvest season results in losses and even production units need to engage untrained labour to manage the season and make the most of it. There have been attempts to develop a mechanical device that can accomplish the tasks of peeling the skin, removing the core, and slicing the fruit, but since it loses a significant amount of fruit pulp, no more development has been made [47,48]. The current writers attempted to employ mechanisation in pineapple processing as part of their academic project, and when the idea was presented to the workers and management, they liked the concept but weren't very interested in moving forward with installing mechanisation and power operated ones [48]. Processing pineapples needs expertise and numerous repetitive hand movements. There were female workers in the processing units too who were involved in pineapple coring and peeling. using modest long knives and cylindrical implements respectively [49].

Farmers play a significant role in the agriculture sector. However, they are encountering a number of occupational traumas and MSDs. For example, repetitive activities, awkward postures, force exertions and more. In addition, most work-related problems have been anticipated to be solved through an ergonomic plan. As a result, these agriculture-related tasks have few negative impacts on people's health. On the other hand, in musculoskeletal areas, physiotherapists have a strong theoretical and practical foundation on which to improve their ergonomic and occupational health skills. The difficulty they face is to broaden the world and apply abilities in the workplace because physiotherapy as a profession plays a significant role in the implementation of ergonomics. Furthermore, micro-ergonomics issues have been seen in school. They have found mismatches between learners' body size, their desks,chairs, heavy school bags and more. As a result, the prevalence of musculoskeletal disorders among school students. Again on the other side, among the office staff who have a causal relationship with computer work. It causes musculoskeletal disorders. With considering the employing some particular tool to use workplace ergonomics and psychosocial factors in office staff with or without reported musculoskeletal pain. Furthermore, "work-related musculoskeletal injuries (WMSIs)" are also common among loco pilots. These ergonomic risk factors have a massive contribution to these injuries. Ergonomics is a multidisciplinary science that focuses on optimising working conditions and job fit. Microergonomics, macroergonomics, environmental ergonomics, cognitive ergonomics, and cultural ergonomics are subfields of ergonomics. A new ergonomic tool for farmers promotes safer work conditions and prevents occupational traumas. Many agricultural instruments can cause injuries, traumas, and MSDs. MSDs are a significant global disorder, as identified by the Finnish Institute of Occupational Health. These diseases are among the most prevalent work-related issues. Agricultural workers often experience musculoskeletal issues due to physical demands, awkward postures, prolonged standing and kneeling, stooping, bending, and repetitive muscle activities, leading to fatigue, illness, and accidents. Additionally, workers' lack of understanding regarding agricultural health and safety might result in life-threatening circumstances. Research and papers confirm the importance of work-related disorders in agriculture. To improve working conditions, ergonomic considerations are necessary for related workers. Ergonomics-based hand tool design ensures optimal conditions. Ergonomics is a human-centred discipline that focuses on improving the quality of life, both at work and in daily life.

Design and Implementation of Work Accessories for Ergonomic Intervention

A hand tool is only considered "ergonomic" when it is designed to fit the task being performed and is intended to be completed, and it fits the hand comfortably without leading to uncomfortable postures, damaging contact pressures, or other safety and health issues [49]. A tool that does not fit the hand or must be handled differently than it was intended (potential misuse), the possibility of injury or muscular strain, and repetitive movements carried out repeatedly or for an extended period of time might exacerbate the risk [50].

Through a business choice, a specific design development for leaf plucking might result in a successful outcome. While workers in small fruit processing facilities (mostly privately owned) perform multiple tasks based on the availability of supplies and their level of expertise in an unpredictable supply-demand production scenario, design development may require a context-specific approach and may involve participatory development. Thus, a thorough investigation was examined to determine the impact of design (work tool) intervention suited for a large working group with corporate decisions for tea-leaf plucking operations [49]. Nearly all fruit processing businesses, especially the small and medium-sized ones, are privately owned. Due to the expensive price, they cannot access the newest technologies. Workers, particularly women workers, are involved in multitasking. Additionally, there is no set distribution of jobs among the employees. The employees carry out a variety of tasks as needed. Design intervention is therefore not a development focused on a single sort of work instrument. The workers use readily available local utility items that they have modified for ease of usage [50].

Conceptually, ergonomically, and technologically, a plucking help was created. It is a finger guard with a blade implanted to make plucking easier and guard against finger anomalies. Its applicability was tested on the employees before being modified in response to input using a participatory approach that included the direct beneficiaries in the development process. The workers not only praised the design's ability to increase productivity but also its value in terms of job comfort [51].

ASSESSMENT OF ERGONOMICS

Assessment Of Ergonomics By Rapid Entire Body Assessment Reba Method

The Justification and Objective of the Rapid Entire Body Assessment Method (REBA)

At Nottingham Hospital (in the United Kingdom), Sue Hignett and Lynn McAtamney created this technique, which was then published in 2000. After identifying and studying almost 600 working postures, a team of ergonomists, physiotherapists, and nurses came up with the solution. The upper limbs (arm, forearm, wrist), trunk, neck, and lower extremities can all be jointly examined with REBA. Additionally, it distinguishes between different kinds of grips and muscular activation. It lists five danger levels, ranging from extremely low to very high [52].

The REBA approach has the following primary benefits:

- It has a good cost-effectiveness ratio.

- It is simple to use. For data collecting, a pen and paper are sufficient, however there are computer programmes that can speed up or facilitate its use.

- The individual score obtained after evaluating every portion of the body is used to identify the ergonomic elements that cause the most conflict [53].

The primary restrictions are:

- It is limited to the examination of specific postures. A group of postures or a series of postures cannot be analysed.

- The evaluator will determine how a task is evaluated. Some of the adopted viewpoints might or might not be looked at.

- It merely assesses the level of effort. Throughout the workday, neither the length of exposure nor the frequency of postures is taken into account [52].

Having the worker's permission to gather the required data is one of the prerequisites of the approach. Each task that will be analysed is seen by the evaluators. Direct observation, videotaping, or capturing pictures are the three methods that observation can be carried out. The goal is to gather information that will enable the procedure to provide outcomes [54].

On the other hand, the approach offers some distinctions from others. It takes into account the worker's lower extremities, which is one of the key variances. Other evaluation techniques, like RULA, do not take this into account. There are no superior or worse procedures; rather, the ones that are used rely on the circumstances and resources of the evaluators. It should be highlighted that when the approach has been published, it is crucial to understand its global application throughout time. The effect of the REBA method on society would be justified by examining how it has been applied over the years [54].

ASSESSMENT OF ERGONOMICS BY RULA

RULA was created to assess how much each worker was exposed to ergonomic risk factors related to upper extremity MSD. The biomechanical and postural load needs of job duties and demands on the neck, trunk, and upper extremities are taken into account by the RULA ergonomic assessment instrument. A one-page worksheet is used to assess the necessary repetition, force, and body position. Scores are entered for each body region in sections A for the arm and wrist and B for the neck and trunk based on the evaluations. Tables on the form are then utilised to assemble the risk factor variables, resulting in a single score that shows the amount of MSD risk, after the data for each location has been gathered and graded [55].

The RULA was created to be simple to operate without the need for expensive tools or a doctorate in ergonomics. The evaluator will give a score for each of the following body regions: upper arm, lower arm, wrist, neck, trunk, and legs using the RULA worksheet [12]. The tables on the form are then utilised to assemble the risk factor variables, resulting in a single score that depicts the amount of MSD risk as indicated below, once the data for each location has been gathered and scored [54].

Preparation of the evaluator

The evaluator should familiarise themselves with the job duties and demands by speaking with the employee being evaluated. They should also observe the employee's postures and movements throughout numerous work cycles. The most challenging postures and job activities (based on worker interviews and first observation), the position maintained for the longest period of time, or the posture with the highest force loads should be considered when choosing the postures to be evaluated. Multiple positions and tasks within the work cycle may typically be examined without using a lot of time and effort thanks to how rapidly the RULA can be completed. Only the right or left side is evaluated at once when using RULA. The assessor might decide whether to evaluate both arms or just one after speaking with the person and watching him or her work. There are two body segment parts on the RULA worksheet, A and B, respectively. The arm and wrist are covered by Section A (left side). The neck, trunk, and legs are covered in Section B (on the right side). This division of the worksheet makes sure that any awkward or restricted neck, trunk, or leg postures that can affect the postures of the arms and wrist are taken into account throughout the assessment [55].

ASSESSMENT OF ERGONOMICS BY OWAS

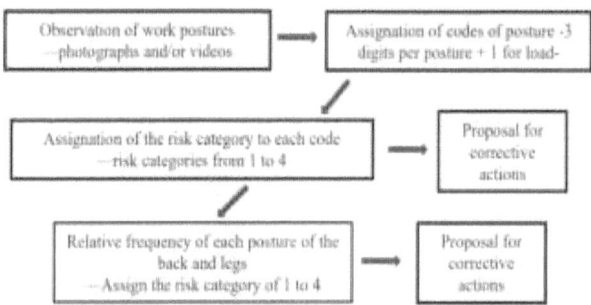

Figure 6: Process flow diagram for submitting an OWAS application

Inception of the OWAS

The OVAKO OY firm, a major European manufacturer of steel bars and profiles, developed the Ovako Working Posture Assessment System (OWAS) in Finland. This technique was employed to assess the workload involved in repairing smelting furnaces) [56].

When the OWAS was first developed, 72 postures were identified by photographing the work postures utilised in various working locations at OVAKO OY. A group of national and international engineers who had been schooled in the method's reliability examined a number of tasks. Two engineers each observed two workers for this purpose over two different work shifts (morning and afternoon). Both groups came to substantially similar conclusions. They then created four danger categories, the first of which was related to standard postures without any suggestions for corrective action. The second and third categories dealt with positions that carried some risk and suggested corrective steps to be implemented in the medium term. Inappropriate postures were classified in the fourth category, and quick corrective action was advised [57].

Methodology of OWAS

The OWAS approach was designed to track how often and how long certain postures were used while performing a task, analyse and assess the situation, and then suggest corrective measures. The most common back postures (4 postures), arms (3 postures), legs (7 postures), and weight of the load handled (3 categories) among employees are all identified by the OWAS. All of this suggests up to 252 different possible combinations. As a result, each posture a worker adopted was given a 4-digit code based on the classification within the prior postures for each body part and the load. Applying the OWAS involved observing the job tasks, codifying the postures, allocating risk categories, and suggesting corrective measures. There are various computer programs that can utilise this technique, allowing for work-time savings, and which have already been used in numerous research [58].

Advantages

It is a well-documented, straightforward strategy that may be applied by staff in a variety of fields (including health, engineering, business, etc.) without the need for specialized training [58].

Limitations

A number of authors failed to distinguish between the right and left upper limbs, evaluate the neck, elbows, and wrists, use a crude posture coding system for the shoulders, take into account repetition or the length of the sequential postures, etc [58].

ASSESSMENT OF ERGONOMICS BY NIOSH

The new NIOSH lifting equation (NLE), which combines the recommended weight limit (RWL) and the lifting index (LI), was released by the National Institute for Occupational Safety and Health (NIOSH) in 1993. NIOSH subsequently released an applications manual with definitions and instructions for using the equations correctly. The RWL is described as "the load value that nearly all healthy workers could perform over a significant period of time (i.e., up to 8 h) without an increased risk of developing lifting-related low back pain (LBP)" for a certain set of task conditions. For a certain lifting task, the lifting index (LI) is calculated as the weight of the load lifted (L) divided by the RWL for that task [59].

The equation has become a widely used tool for determining the physical demands of two-handed manual lifting operations both domestically and abroad. In reality, the new NLE served as the foundation for the European Community's manual lifting requirements. It is anticipated that thousands of people will be gathering data and using the updated NLE with this degree of enthusiasm. However, we are not aware of any prior attempts to ascertain the expected accuracy of the measurement-makers or how those inaccuracies would affect the results and suggestions [56]. A study set out to train a group of non-ergonomists to take the measures required to utilize the NLE and then test their performance roughly two months later. The study's findings should be helpful in evaluating how measurement variability affects the RWL and LI computations as well as in identifying significant training concerns that might have an impact on those measurements [57].

In-depth descriptions of the RWL and LI equations are presented below and were originally published by Waters et al. in 1993 and 1994. The RWL is a multiplicative equation that, in brief, reduces a constant load weight by multipliers that specify the degree of physical stress connected to particular aspects of a lifting operation. The multipliers are calculated using measurements of the load's horizontal (H) and vertical (V) locations relative to the worker's feet, the lift's vertical travel distance (D), the angle of asymmetries between the worker's mid-sagittal line and the load's asymmetry line at the lift-off point (A), the coupling classification (C), and the frequency, rate, and duration of lifting. The multipliers are limited to have a value of 1.0 [58].

RWL = LC * HM * VM * DM * FM * CMLI = L/RWL

RWL: Recommended Weight Limit

LC: Load Constant (a multiplier for different types of lifting activities)

HM: Horizontal Multiplier (a multiplier based on the horizontal distance from the body)

VM: Vertical Multiplier (a multiplier based on the vertical distance from the body)

DM: Distance Multiplier (a multiplier based on the distance from the body)

FM: Frequency Multiplier (a multiplier based on the frequency of lifting)

CMLI: Coupling, Movement, and Lifting Index

L: Load being lifted

Measurement errors will have a variety of effects on the RWL's magnitude because the equation gives varying weights to each of the task elements. For instance, a measurement error of 10 cm in the horizontal distance (H) might cause a maximum inaccuracy in the RWL of roughly 30%. On the other hand, a vertical measurement inaccuracy of 10 cm would only cause a 3% error in the RWL. Comparatively, a 10°

inaccuracy in the asymmetric angle measurement would lead to a maximum error of 3.2% in the RWL [59].

References

1. Scheer SJ, Mital A. Ergonomics. Arch Phys Med Rehabil. 1997 Mar;78(3 Suppl):S36-45.

2. Gupta A, Bhat M, Mohammed T, Bansal N, Gupta G. Ergonomics in dentistry. Int J Clin Pediatr Dent. 2014 Jan;7(1):30-4.

3. Waters TR. Introduction to ergonomics for healthcare workers. Rehabil Nurs. 2010 Sep-Oct;35(5):185-91.

4. Waters TR, Dick RB. Evidence of health risks associated with prolonged standing at work and intervention effectiveness. Rehabil Nurs. 2015 May-Jun;40(3):148-65.

5. Andersen LL, Vinstrup J, Sundstrup E, Skovlund SV, Villadsen E, Thorsen SV. Combined ergonomic exposures and development of musculoskeletal pain in the general working population: A prospective cohort study. Scand J Work Environ Health. 2021 May 01;47(4):287-295.

6. Barnard E, Sheaffer K, Hampton S, Measel ML, Farag A, Shaw C. Ergonomics and Work-Related Musculoskeletal Disorders: Characteristics Among Female Interventionists. Cureus. 2021 Sep;13(9):e18226.

7. Chu PC, Wang TG, Guo YL. Work-related and personal factors in shoulder disorders among electronics workers: findings from an electronics enterprise in Taiwan. BMC Public Health. 2021 Aug 09;21(1):1525.

8. Jin X, Dong Y, Wang F, Jiang P, Zhang Z, He L, Forsman M, Yang L. Prevalence and associated factors of lower extremity musculoskeletal disorders among manufacturing

workers: a cross-sectional study in China. BMJ Open. 2022 Feb 02;12(2):e054969.

9. Menzel NN. Psychosocial factors in musculoskeletal disorders. Crit Care Nurs Clin North Am. 2007 Jun;19(2):145-53.

10. Cornwell L, Doyle H, Stohner M, Hazle C. Work-related musculoskeletal disorders in physical therapists attributable to manual therapy. J Man Manip Ther. 2021 Apr;29(2):92-98.

11. Carayon P, Smith MJ, Haims MC. Work organization, job stress, and work-related musculoskeletal disorders. Hum Factors. 1999 Dec;41(4):644-63

12. Jang TW, Koo JW, Know SC, Song J. Work-related musculoskeletal diseases and the workers compensation. J Korean Med Sci. 2014;29(Suppl.):S18-23. https://doi.org/10.3346/jkms.2014.29.S.S18

13. Punnett L, Wegman DH. Work-related musculoskeletal disorders: the epidemiologic evidence and the debate. J Electromyogr Kinesiol. 2004;14(1):13-23. https://doi.org/10.1016/j.jelekin.2003.09.015

14. Puroila A, Paananen M, Taimela S, Järvelin MR, Karppinen J. Lifestyle factors in adolescence as predictors of number of musculoskeletal pain sites in adulthood: a 17-year follow-up study of a birth cohort. Pain Med. 2015;16(6):1177-85. https://doi.org/10.1111/pme.12697

15. Briggs AM, Cross MJ, Hoy DG, Sánchez-Riera L, Blyth FM, Woolf AD, et al. Musculoskeletal health conditions represent a global threat to healthy aging: a report for the 2015 world health organization world report on ageing and health. Gerontologist. 2016;56(Suppl. 2):S243-55. https://doi.org/10.1093/geront/gnw002

16. Chen X, Mao G, Leng SX. Frailty syndrome: an overview. Clin InterAging. 2014;9:433-41. https://doi.org/10.2147/CIA.S45300

17. Shuai J, Yue P, Li L, Liu F, Wang S. Assessing the effects of an educational program for the prevention of work-related musculoskeletal disorders among school teachers. BMC Public Health. 2014;14:1211. https://doi.org/10.1186/1471-2458-14-1211

18. Nachreiner, F. (1995). Standards for ergonomics principles relating to the design of work systems and to mental workload. *Applied Ergonomics*, *26*(4), 259-263. https://doi.org/10.1016/0003-6870(95)00029-C

19. (2023). Iso.org. https://www.iso.org/obp/ui/#iso:std:iso:6385:ed-2:v1:en

20. ACGIH, 2005. TLVs and BEIs: Threshold limit values for chemical substances and physical agents biological exposure indices. In: American Conference of Governmental Industrial Hygienists, Cincinnati, OH.

21. ACGIH, 2016. Upper limb localized fatigue: TLV(R) physical agents 7th edition documentation. In: American Conference of Governmental Industrial Hygienists, Cincinnati, OH.

22. Auburn Engineers, 2003. ERGO Job Analyzer User's Guide.

23. Buchholz, B., Paquet, V., Punnett, L., Lee, D., Moir, S., 1996. PATH: a work sampling based approach to ergonomic job analysis for construction and other non-repetitive work. Appl. Ergon. 27 (3), 177–187.

24. Burgess-Limerick, R., Straker, L., Pollock, C., Egeskov, R., 2004. Manual tasks risk assessment tool (ManTRA) V 2.0.

In: Human Factors and Ergonomics Society of Australia Annual Conference.

25. Dempsey, P.G., 2019. On the role of ergonomics at the interface between research and practice. In: In: Bagnara, S., Tartaglia, R., Albolino, S., Alexander, T., Fujita, Y. (Eds.), Proceedings of the 20th Congress of the International Ergonomics Association (IEA 2018), vol. 824. Springer Nature, Switzerland, pp. 256–263 Advances in Intelligent Systems and Computing.

26. Dempsey, P.G., McGorry, R.W., Maynard, W.S., 2005. A survey of tools and methods used by certifified professional ergonomists. Appl. Ergon. 36, 489–503.

27. Gallagher, S., Sesek, R.F., Schall Jr., M.C., Huangfu, R., 2017. Development and validation of an easy-to-use risk assessment tool for cumulative low back loading: the Lifting Fatigue Failure Tool (LiFFT). Appl. Ergon. 63, 142–150.

28. Gallagher, S., Schall Jr., M.C., Sesek, R.F., Huangfu, R., 2018. An upper extremity risk assessment tool based on material fatigue failure theory: the Distal Upper Extremity Tool (DUET). Hum. Factors 60 (8), 1146–1162.

29. Fargnoli, M. Design for Safety and Human Factors in Industrial Engineering: A review towards a unifified framework. In Proceedings of the 11th Annual International Conference on Industrial Engineering and Operations Management, Singapore, 7–11 March 2021; pp. 7511–7522.

30. de Galvez, N.; Marsot, J.; Martin, P.; Siadat, A.; Etienne, A. EZID: A new approach to hazard identifification during the design process by analysing energy transfers. *Saf. Sci.* **2017**, *95*, 1–14.

31. Caffaro, F.; Lundqvist, P.; Micheletti Cremasco, M.; Nilsson, K.; Pinzke, S.; Cavallo, E. Machinery-Related

Perceived Risks and Safety Attitudes in Senior Swedish Farmers. *J. Agromed.* **2018**, *23*, 78–91.

32. Gattamelata, D.; Vita, L.; Fargnoli, M. Machinery Safety and Ergonomics: A Case Study Research to Augment Agricultural Tracklaying Tractors' Safety and Usability. *Int. J. Environ. Res. Public Health* **2021**, *18*, 8643

33. D 'zwiarek, M.; Latała, A. Analysis of occupational accidents: Prevention through the use of additional technical safety measures for machinery. *Int. J. Occup. Saf. Ergon.* **2016**, *22*, 186–192.

34. Vigoroso, L.; Caffaro, F.; Micheletti Cremasco, M.; Cavallo, E. Improving Tractor Safety: A Comparison between the Usability of a Conventional and Enhanced Rear-Mounted Foldable ROPS (FROPS). *Int. J. Environ. Res. Public Health* **2022**, *19*, 10195.

35. . Szeto GP, Tsui MM, Sze WW, et al. Issues about home computer workstation and primary school children in Hong Kong: a pilot study. *Work*. 2014;48:485–493. doi:10.3233/WOR-131810.

36. Ryan C, Lewis JM. Computer and internet use in the United States: 2015. Unites states Census Bureau. Available at: https://www.census.gov/content/dam/ Census/library/publications/2017/acs/acs-37.pdf; 2017. Accessed 10.17.20.

37. BLS.gov. Ability to work from home: evidence from two surveys and implications for the labor market in the COVID-19 pandemic. Available at: https://www.bls.gov/opub/mlr/2020/article/ability-to-work-from-home.htm; 2020 Accessed 10.14.20.

38. Bayern M. 85% of businesses will increase remote work after COVID-19 despite security concerns. Available at:

https://www.techrepublic.com/article/84-of-businesses-will-increase-remote-work-after-covid-19-despite-securityconcerns/; 2020 Accessed 10.14.20.

39. Tridandapani S, Holl G, Canon CL. Rapid deployment of home PACS workstations to enable social distancing in the coronavirus disease (COVID-19) era. *AJR Am J Roentgenol*. 2020;215:1351–1353. doi:10.2214/AJR.20.23495.

40. Wong M. Stanford research provides a snapshot of a new working-from-home economy. *Stanford News*. 2020. Available at:. https://news.stanford.edu/2020/06/29/snapshot-new-working-home-economy . Accessed 10.14.20.

41. Fewster KM, Riddell MF, Kadam S, et al. The need to accommodate monitor height changes between sitting and standing. *Ergonomics*. 2019;62:1515–1523. doi:10.1080/00140139.2019.1674931.

42. Kaliniene G, Ustinaviciene R, Skermiene L, et al. Associations between neck musculoskeletal complaints and work related factors among public service computer workers in Kunas. *Int J Occup Med Environ J Health*. 2014;26:670–681. doi:10.2478/s13382-013-0141-z.

43. Armstrong, T.J., Foulke, J.A., Bradley, S.J., and Golstein, S.A. (1982). Investigation of cumulative trauma disorders in a poultry processing plant. *American Industrial Hygiene Association Journal, 43*(2), 103–116.

44. Bobjer, O. (1989). Ergonomic knives. In A. Mital (Ed.), *Advances in industrial ergonomics and safety I* (pp. 291–298). London, UK: Taylor and Francis.

45. Fraser, T.M. (1980). *Ergonomic principles in the design of hand tools* [Occupational Safety and Health Series, 9]. Geneva, Switzerland: International Labour Office.

46. Gjessing, C.C., Schoenborn, T.F., and Cohen, A. (Eds.). (1994). *Participatory ergonomics interventions in meatpacking plants*. Cincinnati, OH, USA: National Institute of Occupational Safety and Health, U.S. Department of Health and Human Services.

47. D. Chakrabarti, Design Ergonomics: need and role", Udyog Pragati, 25, (2), 2001, 37-44.

48. K. Kogi, Ergonomics and Technology transfer into small and medium-sized enterprises, Proceedings of the 13th Triennial conference of the IEA, Tampere, Finland,.7, 1997, 638-640.

49. L.P. Gite, and. B.G. Yadav, Optimum handle height for a push-pull type manually-operated dry land weeder, Ergonomics 33 (12), 1990, 1487–1494.

50. N. Bhattacharyya, S.C. Baruah, R. Borah, P.Bhagawati, Ergonomic assessment of postures assumed by workers in tea cultivation, Proceedings of Interantional conference on HWWE'05 held in IIT, Guwahati, 2005.

51. National Institute for Occupational Safety and Health (NIOSH), Ahmedabad, India, 2010, Report on: Stress at work

52. Hignett S., Mcatamney L. Rapid entire body assessment (REBA) *Appl. Ergon.* 2000;**31**:201–205. doi: 10.1016/S0003-6870(99)00039-3.

53. Karhu O., Kansi P., Kuorinka I. Correcting working postures in industry: A practical method for analysis. *Appl. Ergon.* 1977;**8**:199–201. doi: 10.1016/0003-6870(77)90164-8.

54. Corlett E., Madeley S., Manenica I. Posture targetting: A technique for recording working postures. *Ergonomics.* 1979;**22**:357–366. doi: 10.1080/00140137908924619.

55. *A Step-by-Step Guide Rapid Upper Limb Assessment (RULA)*. (n.d.). https://ergo-plus.com/wp-content/uploads/RULA-A-Step-by-Step-Guide1.pdf

56. Waters, T., Baron, S., and Kemmlert, K. (1998). Accuracy of measurements for the revised NIOSH lifting equation. *Applied Ergonomics*, *29*(6), 433-438. https://doi.org/10.1016/S0003-6870(98)00015-5

57. EU-OSHA (European Agency for Safety and Health at Work). Prevención de los trastornos musculoesqueléticos de origen laboral 2000. https://osha.europa.eu/es/tools and-publications/publications/factsheets/4. Accessed May 20, 2016.

58. EU-OSHA (European Agency for Safety and Health at Work). Introducción a los trastornos musculoesqueléticos de origen laboral 2007. https://osha.europa.eu/es/tools and-publications/publications/factsheets/71. Accessed May 20, 2016.

59. EU-OSHA (European Agency for Safety and Health at Work). OSH in figures: Work-related musculoskeletal disorders in the EU – Facts and figures 2010. Edited by European Agency for Safety and Health at Work (EU OSHA). European Risk Observatory Report, 11 – 26, Luxembourg. https://osha.europa.eu/es/tools-and-publications/ publications/reports/TERO09009ENC. Accessed May 20, 2016

Chapter 3:

Common Occupation Related MSDs And Their Management

A broad spectrum of inflammatory and degenerative illnesses and disorders are referred to as work-related musculoskeletal ailments (Figure 7). These illnesses can affect the neck, shoulders, elbows, forearms, wrists, and hands, causing discomfort and functional impairment. Work-Related Upper Limb Disorders (WRULD), implies a group of musculoskeletal disorders that affect the upper limbs, including the neck, shoulders, arms, wrists, and hands. WRULDs are often associated with repetitive motions, awkward postures, and other ergonomic factors in the workplace. They can cause pain, discomfort, and functional impairment, impacting an individual's ability to perform tasks related to work and daily life [1,2]. When work-related activities and situations significantly contribute to a disorder's onset or aggravation but do not account for all of the factors that cause it, the World Health Assembly recognises that the disorder is work-related (World Health Organisation, 1985). Pathological groupings involving tendons, nerves, muscles, circulation, joints, and bursae can be used to classify WRULDs in general [1,3].

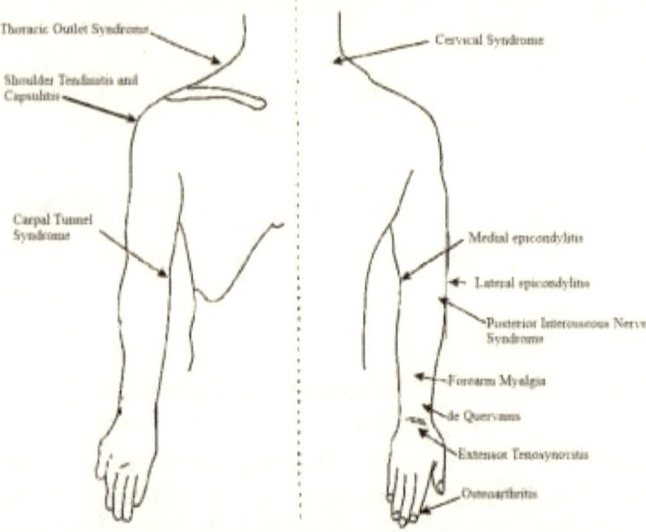

Figure 7: Common Work-Related inflammatory and degenerative illnesses and disorders

There isn't currently a consistent method in place for evaluating WRULDs between or within European Union member states. Recently, criteria were created in the Netherlands and the UK. Each member state's evaluation systems contain a classification for musculoskeletal diseases that lack a clear diagnosis or pathology but nonetheless manifest as pain, discomfort, or functional impairment in the patient [2,3]. It is evident from data sources in the UK that over 50% of patients that arrive with upper limb pain are categorised as non-specific. It is said that distinct sets of information were employed by doctors and researchers to create the assessment criteria for diseases. This has caused considerable misunderstanding. Furthermore, it is still unclear how symptoms, injury reporting, functional impairment, and disability are related. Research goals still include figuring out these connections, documenting the medical natural history of illnesses, and creating standardised criteria [1,2].

Causes of neck and upper limb musculoskeletal diseases caused by job

The body reacts to the dosage in a variety of physiological and biomechanical ways, including increased circulation, localised muscular weariness, and others. The capacity to handle subsequent answers may get better or worse depending on the response. A succession of reactions may further limit the capacity if there is not enough time to allow for bodily tissue regeneration. This cycle of accumulation might go on until some sort of structural tissue distortion happens [1,2].

Others have created models that claim a connection exists between capacity and job activity. When capacity is reduced, less work may be done, and this less work may be enough to give the worker's capacity time to recover. Worker activity is frequently defined as motions and exerted forces that cause the body to produce internal forces. However, the manner in which work is organized (work organisation factors) and the ideas or beliefs that employees have about how work is organized (psychosocial work factors) are what determine the working environment [3].

The development of work-related musculoskeletal illnesses affecting the neck and upper limbs is linked to work organization and psychological work variables, according to reasonable theories and empirical data. The manner the task is done may change depending on the individual worker's anthropometry, level of physical fitness, age, gender, and medical history. Together, these elements may have an impact on the duration, intensity, and frequency of a worker's exposure to working positions, motions, and pressures. All soft tissues, comprising muscle, tendon, ligament, fascia, which is synovia, cartilage, and nerves, are acknowledged to fail in the presence of adequate stress (National Research Council, 1999). Activities performed for work, everyday life, and enjoyment may frequently subject the body to biomechanical stresses that are close to the mechanical limitations of soft tissue [4].

Consideration has been given to ligatures, the connective tissue structures that unite muscle to bone or fascia, and tendon sheaths, which are made of a synovial membrane and shield tendons from mechanical friction as they cross joints. The tendons can get inflamed when they are repeatedly loaded for two different causes. The uniaxial tension forces produced or transferred to the muscle are the primary source of the first, which is increased friction. The second is the transverse reaction forces at the tendon's crossing of nearby hard as well as soft structures such as bursae, pulleys, and retinaculae [4,5]. This happens at the limits of a person's range of motion or when uncomfortable postures are taken. The rubbing of the tendon and the surfaces next to it might be a contributing factor in the development of tendon surface degeneration. For a variety of musculoskeletal conditions, the potential link between local mechanical pressure and the start of nerve injury in the upper limbs has been examined. For instance, improperly constructed instruments and handles can put a direct mechanical strain on the hand's tissues. Numerous weak spots on the palmar part of the hand can be directly compressed by external forces, which might impair the transit of nerve signals, change the structure of the nerve, and perhaps result in ischemia consequences [5].

In a dose-responsive way, non-neutral wrist and forearm postures, as well as force application at the fingers, increase extraneural pressure in the carpal tunnel. These pressures are in line with the degree of disrupted intraneural microvascular blood flow. Inhibiting intraneural capillary flow, axonal transportation, and nerve function, as well as causing endoneurial oedema due to higher intrafascicular pressure and myelin displacement, are all effects of elevated pressures surrounding the nerve. Extraneural pressure can have consequences on nerve structure and function within minutes, and effects on intraneural blood flow can be seen hours after a release of extraneural pressure that was sustained for two hours. Acute effects often recover quickly, but persistent or extremely high pressure might have permanent consequences [6].

Although the pathophysiological mechanism underlying a vibration-induced neuropathy is not fully known, working with vibrating hand tools at work may result in long-term nerve damage. The peripheral nervous system exhibits intraneural oedema, morphological alterations in myelinated and unmyelinated nerve fibres, and also functional abnormalities in both the nerve fibres and non-neuronal cells. These findings are supported by animal models and human biopsy tests. The most typical sign of musculoskeletal problems is muscle discomfort. Chemical impulses from a musculoskeletal problem, both painful and not unpleasant, may make the affected tissues more sensitive. This sensitization has been observed in patients who have chronic musculoskeletal issues and persistent symptoms, and it is likely significant in relation to many work-related musculoskeletal illnesses [7].

Long-term contact with hand-transmitted vibration through powered equipment or processes has been linked to changes in the vascular systems in the upper limbs. A secondary manifestation of Raynaud's phenomenon known as the vibration-induced white finger is the vascular changes that cause finger blanching. In experimental animal investigations or studies of human hands, vascular changes caused by exposure to vibration at different frequencies, acceleration magnitudes, and durations have been described. Additionally, it has been demonstrated that the onset of an acute vibration exposure of 125 Hz causes an instantaneous restriction in vascular flow and that these vasomotor effects last when the vibration exposure has finished. The amount of vascular flow restriction appears to be influenced by the vibration dosage as a function of both acceleration magnitude and exposure time [8].

Carpal Tunnel Syndrome

A common neurological condition known as Carpal Tunnel Syndrome (CTS) develops if the median nerve, which travels from the forearm into the palm of your hand, is pinched or compressed at the wrist. Numbness, weakness, hand and wrist discomfort, as well as bloated and unusable fingers, are possible symptoms. You might feel the desire to "shake out" the palm or wrist when you first wake up [9]. The carpal tunnel, a constrictive, stiff corridor of ligament and bones near the palm of the hand, is where the middle nerve and the tendons that bend the fingertips travel. The thumb, index, middle, and portion of the ring fingers are all sensed by the median nerve, but the little finger is not. Additionally, it has control over a few tiny muscles at the thumb's base. The tunnel can occasionally become smaller and the median nerve can get compressed due to edema or thickening caused by inflamed tendon lining [10]. The most prevalent and well-known entrapped neuropathy, in which a peripheral nerve of the body is pushed against or crushed, is CTS. Carpal tunnel syndrome can occasionally be treated at home, although recovery could take months. Your doctor may make therapy suggestions. After receiving therapy and at-home care, CTS seldom returns [11].

The Structures within the Carpal Tunnel

The scaphoid as well as trapezium tuberosities radially and the pisiform and hook of the hamate medially define the carpal tunnel, which is located on the proximal palmar wrist. The flexor retinaculum, a dense connective tissue covering these four bony prominences, forms a tunnel through which the lengthy flexor ligaments (flexor digitorum profundus, flexor digitorum superficialis, and flexor pollicis longus) pass, holding the prominences in place during wrist flexion. A significant upper limb peripheral nerve is the median nerve [12]. Through the tunnel between the hand and the wrist, through which it branches, it travels from the anterior part of the forearm to supply the thenar muscles with motor supply and sensory innervation for the palmar surfaces on the thumb, index, middle, and radial half of the ring finger. When the canal narrows and the palmar tendons or tendon sheaths bulge, carpal tunnel syndrome results. The symptoms of altered feeling, which commonly affect the radial three and a half digits, are caused by a canal obstruction impinging on the median nerve. However, the symptoms may proceed to produce wasting and weakness in the thenar muscles, weakening the pinch grasp [13].

Symptoms

The symptoms often develop over time and frequently involve tingling or numbness in the fingers, particularly the thumb, index, and middle fingers. Either of the hands will frequently show symptoms for the first time at night. Typically, the dominant hand was the first to be afflicted and had the worst symptoms. Early signs consist of:

- Nervousness, especially at night
- a sensation of uselessness or swelling in the fingers
- a burning or hurting in the fingertips.

As symptoms increase, individuals may experience:

- Mild to severe discomfort, which can get worse at night.
- Tingling throughout the day, especially when doing specific things like chatting over the phone, reading a book and newspaper, or driving.
- A little hand movement loss
- It could be challenging to handle tiny things or carry out other manual chores if your hands are weak.

The muscles near the base of one's thumb may weaken and/or lose away in chronic and/or untreated situations. Some persons with very acute CTS are unable to differentiate between cold and warmth by touch and may accidentally burn their fingertips [14].

Instead of an issue with the nerve itself, carpal tunnel syndrome frequently results from a combination of conditions that put more pressure around the median nerve and tendons within the carpal tunnel. Sometimes it's impossible to pinpoint a single reason. Potential contributing elements include:

- wrist trauma or injury that results in swelling, such as a fracture or sprain
- imbalance in either the thyroid or the pituitary gland
- various rheumatic conditions, such as rheumatoid arthritis
- difficulties with the wrist joint's mechanics
- Vibrating hand tools being used repeatedly
- during menopause or pregnancy, fluid retention
- growth of a tumor or cyst in the canal
- Sex—women have a three-fold higher risk of developing CTS than males

- diabetes and other metabolic conditions that directly impact the body's neurons and increase their susceptibility to compression
- sleeping on a twisted wrist repeatedly
- Getting older—CTS often only affects adults.

The risk of CTS is not specific to any one profession or sector, however, it may be more common among workers who execute assembly line tasks, such as those in manufacturing, crafting, finishing, cleaning, and meatpacking, than among those who enter data. Many persons with CTS reports have never had these kinds of employment [15].

Diagnosis

To prevent the median nerve from suffering lasting injury, early identification, and therapy are crucial.

- Examination of the body: Your doctor will do a physical examination of the fingers, arms, shoulders, or neck to rule out other disorders that resemble carpal tunnel syndrome and to ascertain if your problems are caused by routine tasks or an underlying disorder. The presence of soreness, swelling, warmth, and discolouration in your wrist will be examined. The strength and appearance of atrophy in the tendons and muscles around the bottom of the hand will also be examined, along with the sensation in your fingers.
- Fractures, arthritis, and disorders that harm the nerves, such as diabetes, can be discovered by routine laboratory testing and X-rays.
- The signs of CTS may manifest during certain wrist exams.
- The median nerve, which runs in the wrist is tapped or compressed by the doctor during the Tinel test. If the test

results in tingling within the fingers or a shock-like sensation, it is positive [16].

o You are required to hold your forearms straight while pointing the tips of your fingers downward and squeezing your hands together for the Phalen, and wrist-flexion, test. Within a minute, the fingertips should start to tingle or become more numb if you have CTS. Additionally, your doctor could urge you to attempt making a motion that causes symptoms.

• The diagnosis of CTSs may be supported by electrodiagnostic testing.

o In a study of nerve conduction, the rate of impulse transmission is gauged. The hand and wrist are covered with electrodes, a little electric shock is delivered, and the rate at which nerve impulses are sent is monitored.

o In order to assess the degree of injury to the median nerve, electromyography involves inserting a small needle into a muscle and seeing electrical activity on a screen.

• Additionally, diagnostic imaging might reveal issues or aid with CTS diagnosis.

o The median nerve might appear to be of abnormal size on ultrasound imaging.

o MRIs can display the architecture of the wrist, but they have not been shown to be very helpful in the diagnosis of carpal tunnel syndrome [17].

Multiple Diagnoses

Neuropathies are the primary differential diagnosis for CTS. Cervical radiculopathies at C6–C7 might resemble sensory symptoms, however, in these situations, the radial nerve's distribution will be affected motorically, impairing wrist flexion and triceps. In addition to other reasons for medial neuropathy, those suffering from neuropathic palmar finger pain should take an ulnar or tiny fibre neuropathy into consideration. Pain itself might be challenging to localise. A T1 radiculopathy may also contribute to thenar muscle waste [18].

Carpal tunnel syndrome risk factors at the individual level

The majority of studies' findings indicate that women are more likely than males to develop carpal tunnel syndrome, with a 1.5 per 1000 annual incidence compared to a 0.5 per 1000 annual incidence for men frequency appears to be influenced by gender as well, with women seeing a peak in frequency between the ages of 45 and 54. The increased risk for carpal tunnel syndrome in pregnant and nursing women, as well as women in their first year of menopause, those taking oral contraceptives or hormone replacement therapy, and oophorectomy, appear to lower the incidence, suggesting that hormonal factors may account for at least some of the gender differences. Carpal tunnel syndrome is highly correlated with body mass index and obesity, with the risk of the disorder rising by 8% for every 1 unit rise in body mass [19].

Management of Carpal Tunnel Syndrome

The first treatment for CTS is to ask the patient to prevent pressurising the carpal tunnel, specially during occupational activities. Hand splinting, regional and systemic steroids, non-steroidal anti-inflammatory medications (NSAIDs), diuretics, ultrasonography, and other conservative measures have all been explored [20].

Wrist bracing

It is very recommended to use a nighttime splint for maintaining the arm in a neutral posture. Interestingly, this approach is not well supported by research, at least according to a review published in 2012 by the Cochrane collaboration, which concluded that despite 19 studies with a total of almost 1200 participants, there was little proof that a nocturnal splint was superior to no therapy in the short term. The safety and efficacy of a single splint design and wearing schedule over others, as well as the superiority of splinting over the application of other non-surgical therapies for CTS, were also evaluated as lacking adequate evidence. However, Piazzini and colleagues found "moderate" evidence of splinting, particularly if worn full-time, in a systematic review that was published in 2007. However, it should be kept in mind it is extremely difficult to conduct a research to thoroughly examine the efficacy of splints given how impossible it is to traditionally "blind" people [21].

NSAIDs and diuretics

Diuretics or non-steroidal anti-inflammatory medications are not specifically recommended by the evidence.

Swallowed corticosteroids

Over two weeks as well as four weeks of follow-up, short-term oral corticosteroids were demonstrated to be useful for the symptomatic management of CTS. However, except in the rarest clinical situations, oral corticosteroids are rarely advised as a treatment alternative due to their toxicities and side effects [22].

Injection of a local corticosteroid

A study by the Cochrane collaboration found that after one month, local corticosteroid injection provided more clinical improvement in symptoms than placebo in 12 studies with 651 participants. However, they discovered inadequate proof of symptom improvement after a month. For up to three months, local corticosteroid injection offered noticeably higher clinical improvement versus oral corticosteroid. Over the course of an 8-week follow-up, there was absolutely no proof that a local injection of corticosteroid improved the clinical result when compared to anti-inflammatories. In comparison to one injection, two local injections of corticosteroid did not significantly improve clinical outcomes [23].

Ultrasound

Over a two-week follow-up period, combined data from two studies with 63 individuals failed to demonstrate any appreciable benefits of ultrasound therapy. However, following seven weeks of ultrasonography (which continued at six months) a different experiment showed a considerable reduction in symptoms [24].

Surgery to relieve the carpal tunnel

For severe instances of CTS, like when there's thenar muscle atrophy or weakening of the thumb opposition, and when conservative therapy has failed, surgery to relieve the tunnel of the wrist is suggested. In Canada, the lateral carpal ligament was initially surgically released in an open procedure in 1924, and after the 1950s, carpal tunnel release (CTR) operation gained widespread acceptance. More than 51,000 CTRs were performed within England in 2012, making it the most popular hand procedure in the UK. Although there is considerable controversy about how "success" can be accurately defined, surgical success rates of 54–75% are often reported [25].

Following carpal tunnel release surgery, going back to work

Despite the prevalence of CTR, there's presently no agreement on the ideal postoperative time course and manner for returning to work. Some studies indicate the length of post-operative illness absence, but the data is inconsistent and frequently leaves out information on a person's typical working hours or schedule [18]. It is important to take into account factors including the requirement for a graded return to work (with modified responsibilities or fewer hours), both worker and employer contentment with job performance, and pain or discomfort at work.

Individual traits have been proven to be independently related to a delayed return to work, including older age, female gender, being overweight, co-occurring musculoskeletal illnesses, and poorer educational attainment. Naturally, aspects related to the patient's return to work, such as the patient's kind of profession, are also crucial [26].

People who must restart physical labour, repetitive motions, or ergonomic pressures all take longer to get back to work than those who are not affected by these elements at work. It has also been discovered that pre- and post-operative clinical factors play a role, so those who report the most severe pre-operative symptoms, those who require pre-operative sick leave, those who require bilateral surgery, those who undergo open rather than endoscopic procedures, and those who report post-operative pain as well as scar tenderness all have a slower return to work. Psychological and psychological issues that might affect return to work include poorer mental wellness, reduced self-efficacy, unhappiness with surgery, poor job security, poor coworker support, higher job expectations, and lesser workplace control [27].

Rehabilitation

The term "physical therapy," also known as "physiotherapy," is derived from the Greek words "fysis," which means "nature," and "therapia," which means "treatment." It combines a number of elements designed to prevent and treat diseases using both natural (such as the sun, sea, recuperation mud, water, and movement) and artificial elements (such as electricity, ultrasound, artificial light, laser rays, magnetic field, etc.). Their impact lessens pain, promotes healing processes, expands the range of motion, engages immune systems, and enhances biochemical efficiency [28].

In comparison to other treatments, physical therapy is less expensive, non-invasive, and simple to use. The most prevalent compressive mononeuropathy in the upper limb is carpal tunnel syndrome (CTS). The earliest available time should be used to begin CTS treatment. Appropriate physiotherapy rehabilitation programs may often restore the functioning of the damaged hand in circumstances when abnormalities in the anatomy of the carpal canal are absent [29].

Depending on the illness stage, the intensity of the symptoms, the objective changes that have been demonstrated, the distinctive features of the patient, and any underlying conditions, the best combination of physical variables and kinesiotherapy is sought. Physiotherapy sessions typically last for 10 days and can be repeated numerous times with a 2- to 4-week rest in between. A few of the subsequent physical characteristics are often taken into account in therapeutic courses for CTS [28-30].

1. Depending on the illness stage, the extent of the signs, the selectivity of the treated tissue due to their water percentage, and the patient's personal tolerance, exogenous heat through paraffin or endogenous heat via ultra-high frequency treatment (UHFT) is utilised. On the anatomical extension between the carpal canal as well as the palm, paraffin is applied for 15 to 20 minutes at a temperature of around 50 °C. UHFT is administered in the range of oligothermic doses (low to moderate heat feeling) to athermic doses (absence of heat sensation) [29]. Thermal therapies are utilised to enhance nerve transmission and trophy, reduce paresthesia, reduce stiffness, and analgesia. Additionally, they might be utilized as

a warm-up treatment for later ultraphonophoresis. Targeted radiofrequency treatment (Tekar therapy), a procedure whereby high-frequency electromagnetic waves generate warmth in depth, is an additional heat factor substitute. This therapy's underlying idea is sometimes referred to as long-wave diathermy. It reduces inflammation and quickens the process of tissue repair [31].

2. Laser therapy is employed to alleviate pain and paresthesia symptomatically. A number of the first treatments for CTS that the FDA has approved is laser therapy. It is suitable to utilize either low- or intense laser rays with the accompanying dosing regimen.

3. The fibrinolytic, anti-inflammatory, and anti-irritant effects of ultrasound are used in ultrasound treatment. The use of a low-frequency transducer for deeper impact or a high-frequency one for surface effect is applied to the projection within the carpal canal. The treatment is known as ultraphonophoresis when nonsteroidal anti-inflammatory medicines (NSAIDs) are employed in the contact gel; the dose is lower (0.4-0.6 W/cm2) and the time is shorter (6-8 minutes). After a surgical operation, a similar technique is routinely done. Due to their fibrinolytic impact, other treatments for skin scars are favored in adhesions [32].

4. To increase oxidative processes and tissue trophic responses, and inhibit oxidative activity, One of the contentious physical elements in the complicated treatment of CTS is magnetotherapy, which is contraindicated in patients with pacemakers.

5. Iontophoresis is utilized to combine the galvanic and low-frequency current's analgesic impact with potassium iodide's fibrinolytic action. The process involves applying a 5%

solution containing potassium iodide to the hydrophile cushion within the negative electrode [33].

6. Another method for easing CTS discomfort is acupuncture. Its anesthetic effect is equivalent to topical corticosteroid treatment when appropriately applied.

7. Another of the non-invasive and scientifically supported physical techniques to treating CTS is shockwave therapy (SWT). In the ligamentum carpi transversalis, SWT is used. There are 4-6 treatments total in the therapeutic regimen, with 1-2 procedures every week. When the CTS is linked to occupational overload and is seen in young patients or in the early stages of the illness.

8. To stop the injured hand from making active motions, immobilization is advised. There will be very little stress within the carpal canal since the wrist remains in a neutral posture.

For the same reason, the interphalangeal and carpometacarpal joints are locked in a mild flexion.

9. Kinesiotherapy, particularly mechanotherapy, aids in recovering motor function, enhancing nervous system excitability and conduction, and preserving the trophy within the thenar's paretic muscles. A mild, attentive massage which should be given every day might affect muscle hypotrophy [34].

Ergonomic interventions

There are surgical and nonsurgical options for CTS therapy. Surgery is often recommended for those with severe CTS who exhibit ongoing symptoms, substantial sensory disruption, or both the motor weakness and sensory impairment. Those who experience mild to moderate CTS intermittent symptoms are given non-surgical therapies. While waiting for carpal tunnel release (CTR), non-surgical therapies may potentially be employed as a temporary fix. Numerous interventions, including ergonomic modification of tools or positioning (such as ergonomic keyboards and handles), splinting, ultrasound for therapy, workouts, yoga, oral medication, vitamins, and complementary therapies are among the alternatives to surgery for the treatment of CTS. Uncertainty surrounds their efficacy in CTS treatment. The above-mentioned surgical treatment of CTS provides symptom alleviation by enlarging the carpal tunnel. Different pathophysiological elements of CTS must be addressed for non-surgical therapies to be effective [35].

The Back Safety (BS) program, which is utilized in a number of nations like Germany, Austria, Hungary, Sweden, Canada as well, Iran, the United States, the Netherlands, Norway, Spain, and the United Kingdom, is the most commonly used patient education program for spine illnesses. The BS program has a learning and skill component that includes activities where patients are taught in groups under the supervision of an orthopedic surgeon or medical professional [36].

The teaching component of BS is predicated on the idea that patients are more at risk and experience more pain than required since they lack knowledge regarding their condition and are unfamiliar with concepts like stress and body mechanics. Therefore, BS initiatives seek to lower the risk of back issues by raising patient education, which in turn alters patient behavior by encouraging the adoption of safe lifting techniques and healthy body posture at work [37].

BS courses often contain educational interventions where participants learn about the anatomy and function of their back, mechanical strain, and posture in addition to receiving isometric exercise regimens. In addition, BS may cover body mechanics, transfer of patient techniques, stretching and strengthening recommendations, instructional handouts, details about back care, being physically fit, resting to avoid pain, performing analgesic exercises, daily activity, seated posture, sitting posture, alternate positions of the body throughout everyday tasks, home exercises, activities to increase lumbar spine mobility, exercises for strengthening the abdominal muscles and the back muscles, as well as details on back pain [38].

Back to School initiatives are well-liked because they follow educational concepts, can be planned for groups, don't need pricey or sophisticated technology, and the participants typically look forward to the sessions. Thus, BS initiatives provide a practical, efficient, and affordable intervention [39]. Determining what defines healthy body posture is the hardest part. However, a biomechanical measuring procedure may be used to evaluate changes in body position. Passive treatments are the foundation of most medical procedures for chronic low back pain in Hungary. Despite the numerous studies and several worldwide guidelines that support the adoption of such tactics, only around 20% of cLBP sufferers are treated with active medications. Passive therapy has been shown to be unsuccessful in treating people with chronic lower back pain and in preventing new back disorders [40].

How the treatment could operate

In order to allow the most room inside the carpal tunnel and to prevent repeatedly or continuously putting the wrist into flexion or extension, ergonomic positioning and equipment in treating CTS positions the hand in a neutral position (Hagberg 1992). For instance, changing the angle on a tool handle and keyboard can do this [41]. By adopting robotic management of vibrating machinery, insulating tool handles, or wearing gloves, treatments can decrease or even eliminate the hand's exposure to vibration. To avoid extended static retention of the weight use the arm, forearm, and hand, further ergonomic solutions include the employing of forearm supports and workspace modifications (Herbert 2000).

The number of jobs that need keyboard and mouse use is rising everywhere, especially in computerised communications sectors. Despite cross-sectional and prospective research, there is still some uncertainty regarding the connection between CTS and keyboard and mouse usage [42].

Tendinitis And Tenosynovitis

Tendinitis

Tendons are strong, intricate connective structures that let muscles push against bones to move joints. The majority of their dry weight is made up of type I collagen organised in parallel fibres, with the remaining 20% to 30% consisting of minor components such proteoglycans, glycosaminoglycans, and additional collagens [43].

Although tendons' structure and other features give them exceptional tensile strength and the ability to carry stress from muscle to bone, a number of these same features also have a negative impact on their ability to repair. As a result, many visits to family care and sports medicine doctors are for chronic tendon issues, such as tendonitis and tendinopathies [44].

Tenosynovitis is an inflammation that affects the tendon and its sheath, whereas tendinitis is an inflammation of the tendon itself. Tendinosis is the non-inflamed degradation of the bundles of collagen that make up the tendon tissue. It is crucial to comprehend the many kinds of tendons in order to distinguish between these entities. Synovial sheaths, which reduce the frictional forces experienced during tendon mobility, are frequently present on tendons with changed directional courses, those bound by tunnels, and those bound by retinacula. Sheaths are frequently absent from linear tendon tissues. The Achilles tendon isn't sheathed, although its posterior tibial tendon and peroneal tendons are among the often damaged tendons of the foot and ankle. Instead, a delicate vascular layer called the paratenon surrounds the Achilles tendon. A layer rich in mucopolysaccharides lies beneath this, allowing the Achilles substantial flexibility of mobility [45].

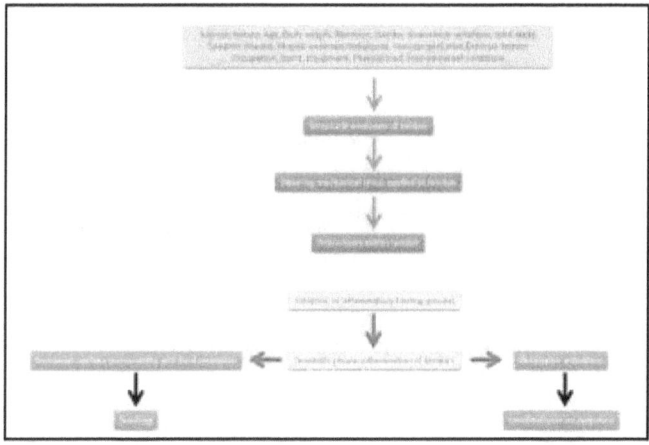

Figure 8: The Pathogenesis and consequence of Tendinitis

Etiology

The majority of long-term tendon injuries are caused by a confluence of intrinsic and extrinsic causes.

Extrinsic Elements

The common consensus is that one of the primary contributors to chronic tendinopathy is mechanical stress. It may be further divided into subcategories, such as longer duration, more frequent occurrences, and higher intensity, as well as technical faults. Other extrinsic variables, such as incorrect form, unsuitable footwear—from running shoes to work tools—and a lack of protective clothing, also worsen the effects of mechanical stress [46].

<u>Intrinsic Elements</u>

Anatomical, aging-related, and systemic variables are examples of intrinsic variables that predispose someone to the development of chronic tendinopathies. Malalignment, stiffness, eccentric muscular usage, and muscle weakness or imbalance are examples of anatomical variables. This is frequently connected to chronic tendinopathies in younger individuals, along with mechanical overload tendencies. Tendon degradation, a lowered healing response, an increase in tendon stiffness, and a decrease in tendon vascularity are age-related variables that affect chronic tendinopathies. Diabetes mellitus, overweight, tobacco use, and inflammatory enthesopathies are examples of systemic causes [44-47].

Tenosynovitis

The inflammation of the fluid-filled synovium inside the tendon sheath is referred to as tenosynovitis. Depending on the cause, it frequently presents as discomfort, swelling, and contractures. The hand, wrist, and foot are the most often affected joints, while the disorder may impact every tendon in the human body with a sheath. The doctor can grasp the pathogenesis, therapy, and problems with a fundamental awareness of the tendon structure. The hand provides a clear illustration of the tendon structure and its link to the tendon sheath [48].

The complex arrangement of tendons in the hand enables the hand's gripping, grasping, and fine motor function.

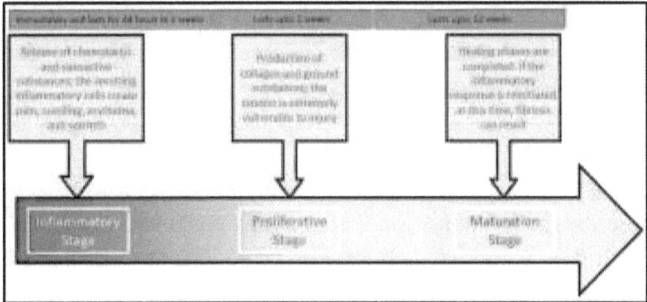

Figure 9: The pathophysiology of Tenosynovitis and its stages of pathological process

The following roles are performed by the tendon sheath:

- The synovial fluid hydrates the tendon and creates a low-friction environment that enables smooth tendon gliding and lessens friction-related tendon wear and strain.

- The fibrous sheath gives the tendon anchor points to prevent "bowstringing." To avoid the tendons from bending when the fingers are flexed, they assist in anchoring the tendons to the bone plane between the phalanges and interphalangeal joints in the hand [49].

Both infectious and non-infectious conditions can result in tenosynovitis. Idiopathic, autoimmune, and overuse are examples of non-infectious causes.

Autoimmune:

Tenosynovitis and rheumatoid arthritis are strongly associated, and tenosynovitis radiological characteristics can be seen in as many as 87% of patients with this condition on MRI. Synovial linings are particularly susceptible to rheumatoid arthritis. Given the large synovial component of the tendon sheath, the tendon sheath may play a crucial part in the development of the disease and the manifestation of the patient's symptoms.

Although this has been demonstrated in a mouse trial, it has not yet been established in people. Another often-related autoimmune disorder is psoriasis [50].

Overuse:

Overuse syndrome or repetitive strain injury are terms used to describe the inflammation within the synovial sheath that can result from repetitive motions. Long durations of computer use that cause stress on the fingers, wrist, and forearm are a common example. Tenosynovitis and tendon discomfort are both increased by any extended, repeated motions [51].

Idiopathic:

Idiopathic tenosynovitis is a form of the disease in which there is no known etiology.

Infective:

The proliferation of infectious microorganisms inside the tendon sheaths results in infectious tenosynovitis. They can spread from nearby or far-off illnesses or by direct injection from wounds to the sheaths. Staphylococcus aureus (40 for 75%), MRSA (29%), Staphylococcus epidermidis, a beta-hemolytic Streptococcus, *P. aeruginosa*, Eikinella during human bites, and *Pasturella multocida* with animal bites are among the prevalent organisms detected in infective tenosynovitis [52].

Tenosynovitis causes can be assessed and distinguished from one another through laboratory testing. It's not always essential, though. It may be important to consider observations of high WBC, bacteremia, and culture when considering infectious causes of tenosynovitis. Specific indicators may show up in autoinflammatory illnesses to help with diagnosis. When infection or inflammation is detected, microscopic analysis can aid further in separating crystalline pathology from those conditions. While not always essential, imaging analysis is useful in the diagnosis of tenosynovitis. Plain film radiographs frequently reveal synovial membrane calcifications or, sometimes, periosteal response, which suggests inflammation; nonetheless, they may be completely clear. Although computed tomography can be helpful for spotting skeletal abnormalities such as bony erosions and structural anomalies, it has limited sensitivity to soft tissue conditions like synovitis and tenosynovitis [53].

In the hands, which can show echotexture alterations in 15% of tendons as well as blurring in the tendon borders in 62%, ultrasound frequently adds diagnostic value. In addition, 44% of fingers had tendon thickening evident, 6% had sheath cysts, and 4% had other abnormalities in the metacarpophalangeal joints. Further assessment using MRI is a possibility when ultrasonography is constrained or when further precise evaluation is necessary [54]. In situations involving infectious etiologies for abscess visualisation, contrast should be taken into account. In instances of de Quervain tenosynovitis, MRI findings of tenosynovitis often show peri-tendinous edema and increased thickness of both the Extensor Brevis Longus (EBL) and abductor Pollicis Longus (APL) tendon. The bone marrow signal can grow more pronounced in rheumatoid arthritis before tenosynovitis symptoms appear. Fluid collections that exhibit enhancement may be the beginning of an abscess [55].

When empiric treatment is required, broad-spectrum antibiotics like vancomycin at the dosage of 15 to 20 mg/kg/dose each 8 to 12 hours in a third-generation cephalosporin that 1 to 2 g IV every 24 hours are taken into consideration and may improve outcomes for infectious tenosynovitis. The length of time depends on the clinical symptoms, the presence of absence of bacteremia, and the infection's origin. Patients with stage 1 infection may undergo sheath irrigation, with catheter-directed treatment producing better results than open irrigation. Debridement will probably be necessary for individuals who have stage 2 or stage 3 infections [56]. Depending on the etiology, non-infectious forms of tenosynovitis are treated in different ways, although for many, non-steroidal anti-inflammatory medications like naproxen are used conservatively. Activity moderation, splinting, and injections of glucocorticoids might also be used as additional first-line treatments. Patients who fail a trial of NSAIDs may also benefit from disease-modifying antirheumatic medications (DMARDs), such as glucocorticoids. Even with conservative treatment, following three to six months of disease advancement, surgery could be required. Decompression of the afflicted tendon as well as the removal of inflammatory tissues are also possible surgical interventions [57].

Treatment of tenosynovitis

Tenosynovitis, which causes excruciating tendon sheath inflammations, is particularly prevalent in the hands and feet. Usually, the discomfort subsides after some time of resting the inflamed region. Physiotherapy, injections, or - if that doesn't work - surgery can assist if the symptoms don't go away. The tendons and tendon sheaths involved may swell up as a result of repetitive motions or specific strains. For instance, if you write using a computer and smartphone a lot, this might occur within the fingers or wrists. This type of inflammation, known as tenosynovitis, can also cause swelling, which makes it difficult to move the fingers. If you exert too much stress on the ankle joints, such as by walking far distances without enough preparation, it may also happen [58].

After conservative therapy, which includes physiotherapy, medications, and immobilisation (keeping the afflicted region immobile), the inflammation frequently already goes away. It may be a good idea to make modifications to the workplace if the inflammation has been brought about by a work-related activity, such as switching into an ergonomic mouse or computer use. Ask for assistance if you're unsure if making adjustments will be beneficial, such as from a health care professional [57,59].

Respite from pain and immobilisation:

Resting the afflicted region is crucial, and you should especially refrain from the motions that first triggered the inflammation. You might need to obtain a sick note via the physician and take the day off work to accomplish this. If you can't totally avoid a certain movement, attempt to execute it less frequently or with less vigor. A plaster cast, constricted bandage, or specialized orthopaedic brace might also be beneficial, for example, by stabilizing the wrist or thumb. Non-steroidal anti-inflammatory medicines (NSAIDs), which reduce inflammation, can also be ingested or administered topically, especially if the inflamed region feels even when it's not being moved. These drugs lessen edema and inflammation while also relieving pain. Many claim that chilling the afflicted region relieves pain, however, heat may also be used. One may experiment on oneself to find what's most effective for you when administering cold or heat [60].

Exercise and massage treatment:

Movement is not restricted, despite the need to rest the afflicted area of the body. For instance, you might try to lessen the discomfort by doing stretching or mobilisation exercises if the tenosynovitis prevents you from moving the finger or wrist adequately. Additionally helpful are massages or other therapies offered by a physiotherapy office. Electrical nerve stimulation through the skin (TENS) or acupuncture may also be used to treat tenosynovitis [61].

Injections of anaesthetic and steroid medications:

Doctors will occasionally use injections to try to lessen the symptoms of very chronic tenosynovitis. Most frequently, an anaesthetic called lidocaine and a corticosteroid is injected straight into the inflammatory region. Some tendons pass through a small tunnel comprised of bones and ligaments, such as those found in the wrists and fingers. They have tendon sheaths to keep them safe. The tendon may find it challenging or even impossible to move into the tendon sheath as a result of the swelling associated with tenosynovitis. Stenosing tenosynovitis is the medical word for this condition. Here, too, conservative treatment modalities including rest, physiotherapy, and painkillers can be beneficial.

The Carpal Tunnel is a sheath surrounded confined area that can be operated in case of increasing or pain refractory to any drugs. The tissue or sheath may be surgically removed in order to provide more space and relieve the pain [62]. The quick operation is frequently performed in an outpatient environment, so there is typically no need for significant skin incisions. As a result, you can return home the same day. Once the wound has healed, it is crucial to provide the injured area of the body some rest and protection [60-62]. However, that does not imply that you cannot move it. The opposite is true: It's beneficial to stretch the afflicted tendons many times each day, but gently. You may move that area on the body normally again within a few weeks without experiencing any pain. Include any procedures, this one might have negative side effects including infections and issues with wound healing. Additionally, possible side effects include unusual feelings or restricted movement [63].

Rehabilitation of tendonitis and tenosynovitis

In contemporary western countries, tendinopathies are among the most frequent musculoskeletal and sports injuries. For the treatment of tendinopathy, a variety of physiotherapy techniques have been suggested [64].

Eccentric exercise is the most effective method of managing tendinopathy. The three guiding principles of eccentric workouts are load, speed, and frequency of contractions. The three guiding principles of eccentric workouts are load, speed, and frequency of contractions. When eccentric exercise load is raised without considering the patient's symptoms, the outcomes are subpar. Stanish et al. (2000) recommend that to imitate the mechanism of damage, which often happens at rather high velocities, the stress on the tendon ought to be increased with each therapy session. However, eccentric workouts should be carried out slowly to promote tissue repair and prevent the potential for further damage [65].

Speed rotation is below the tendon's elastic limit and produces less harmful heat inside the tendon. The literature has a variety of repetitions and sets. Typically, three sets totaling 15 repetitions are advised. One or two sets are completed each day. For many individuals with tendinopathies, eccentric exercise alone is ineffective. As a consequence, the combination of eccentric training and static stretching exercises is effective in treating tendinopathies [66].

Lower Back Pain And Lumbar Disorders

Vertical lumbosacral, radicular, and referred pain are the three main types of low back pain. Back discomfort in the lumbar, or L1–5 vertebral area, and sacral spine, or S1– sacrococcygeal junction region, is referred to as axial lumbosacral back pain. Leg pain that radiates into an extremity due to nerve or dorsal root ganglion stimulation follows a dermatomal distribution.

Referred pain travels from its origin but follows a non-dermatomal path. The problem of low back pain can be divided into acute (6 weeks), acute (6–12 weeks), and persistent (> 12 weeks) lower back pain as well as being divided by the location of the pain. While most non-chronic patients have acute pain that subsides in 6 weeks with less, 10–40% of individuals experience symptoms that continue longer than 6 weeks. Patients with acute and subacute backaches are treated differently from those with persistent low back pain [67].

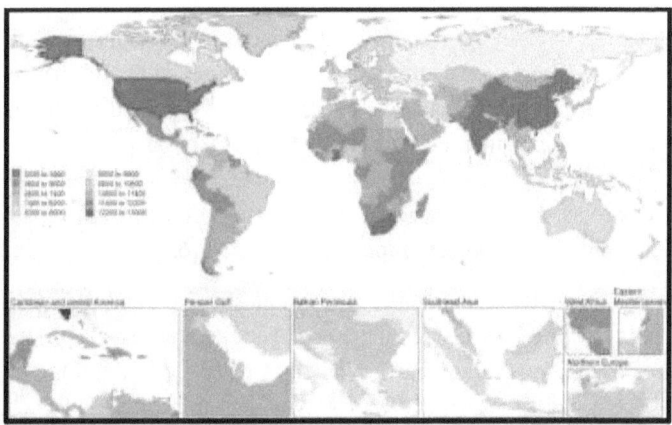

Figure 10: Prevalence of Low Back Pain per 100,000 population in 2019 (country-wise) [60]

The risk that an acute bout if low back pain would turn chronic and incapacitating is the biggest consequence. The prevalence of low back pain and the associated disability is rising. According to the findings of the 2015 Worldwide Cost in Disease research, 60.1 million years of disability worldwide were attributed to low back pain [60]. This represented a rise of 54% from 1990. Most people who have low back pain have brief episodes; however, 28% of individuals develop a chronic handicap, which accounts for 77% of all low back pain-related disabilities. The percentage of people with low back pain who are disabled is higher among those who are working, and this pattern is seen in both low- and middle-income nations [68]. Among the top 5 illnesses restricting activity was low back discomfort, according to a poll of urban people in Zimbabwe. More than 50% of Nigerian peasant farmers who participated in the study reported reducing their labour as a result of low back discomfort. In the US, the yearly immediate expense of backache is thought to be between $50 and $90 billion. It is estimated that low back pain costs society $635 billion yearly in direct medical expenses as well as lost productivity [69].

Unfortunately, a sizable majority of people who suffer from chronic low back pain also have pain in other body regions and have other issues with their physical and mental health. The combined impact of co-morbidity and low back pain is bigger than the individual impacts of either co-morbidity or low back pain. This leads to a greater demand for care and a less effective response to treatment [70].

According to a research that examined data taken from the 2010 National Health Interview Survey (NHIS) from the US, female and older employees were more likely to experience low back discomfort. They also identified additional psychological characteristics as possible risk factors, such as an imbalance between work and family, unfriendly working conditions, and job instability [71].

Evaluation of patients with Low Back Pain

Lower back discomfort has a few distinctive features that need to be clarified. In order to aid in decision-making, the length of the patient's symptoms is used to classify them as either acute, subacute, or chronic low back pain. It's crucial to identify and define the source of the low back discomfort, whether it's axial or radicular. With the use of a particular scale, the degree of pain may be measured. The results can be used to calculate the best, worst, average, and current ratings. Screening inquiries regarding troubling symptoms of constitution (red flags) which could indicate a potential progressive and unstable source of pain, including cancer, infection, trauma, and neurologic deterioration, should be part of the first examination for a patient with lower back pain [72].

Lower back pain may have several causes, but one that should be considered for therapy is a history of infections caused by a recent illness, fever, spinal injection, spinal catheter installation, IV medication usage, immunosuppression, or other concurrent infections. Finally, individuals with bladder and bowel control issues may also have neurologic deterioration because urine retention may result from spinal cord and cauda equina compression, which may then cause urinary and/or faecal incontinence. It is important to assess those who have lower back pain for social or psychological discomfort. An evaluation of past substance addiction, disability benefits, employment status, and depressive symptoms is a sign of such psychological distress [73].

Physical examination in patients with Low Back Pain

A lengthy or quick physical examination is a necessary component of managing low back pain. Vital signs, ambulation status (aides, mobility, and gait), appearance, behaviour, symptoms of anxiety, skin, mood and affect judgement, and mental process are all significant patient data that may be obtained via a routine physical examination. Additionally, a neurological checkup should be carried out, including examining the upper motor neuron reflexes, sensitivity, deep tendon reflexes, and back and lower extremity motor strength. Additionally, individuals with epidural tumours, abscesses, and spinal compression fractures may exhibit localized discomfort upon probing across the spinous processes. The physical exam also includes a number of tests for various conditions. Patrick's test assesses sacroiliac and hip pathologies, each of which is connected to lower back pain [74].

The examiner should gently flex, abduct, and exterior rotate the hip while the patient is supine. Back pain denotes sacroiliac joint disease whereas discomfort in groin suggests hip pathology. A simple leg raise test ought to be performed to rule out any hamstring or lumbar nerve root connection to the lower back discomfort. The examiner should elevate the patient's leg at the heel with the knee straight while they are supine [72-75].

Hip flexion should range from 70° to 90°. The lumbar nerves tense up as a result of this examination. Positive straight leg raises replicate the patient's radicular discomfort, which must radiate through a radicular pattern from the bottom of his back and hip down to his ankle. Hamstring strain is most likely to blame if discomfort is still restricted to one's posterior thigh region. In order to determine whether lower back discomfort is originating from the sacroiliac joints, a Gaenslen's test should be performed, as shown in Figure 11 [75,76].

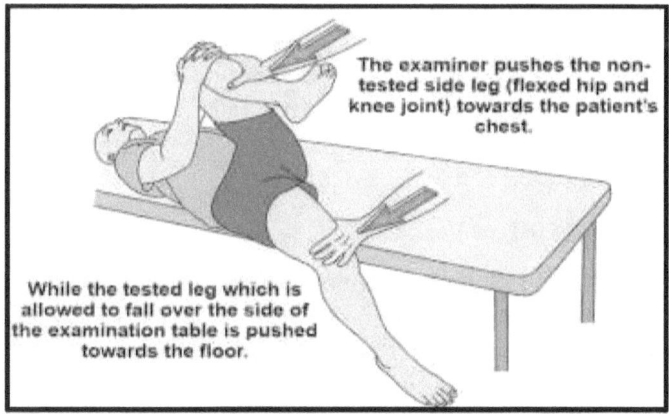

Figure 11: Gaenslen's test is done to diagnose any pathology around sacroiliac joints

Diagnostic Evaluation in Low Back Pain

Diagnostic Tests are done only when necessary for treating lower back pain. Rarely, laboratory tests are required. However, patients with suspected infection or cancer can be evaluated with Erythrocyte Sedimentation Rate (ESR) and/or C-Reactive Protein (CRP) alongside plain radiographs to assess whether further imaging is necessary. Additionally, imaging examinations are only carried out under certain conditions. The majority of people having lower back pain that has been present for less than four weeks do not need Magnetic Resonance Imaging (MRI). Imaging should only be done when there are significant or developing neurologic impairments or when a major neurologic condition is strongly suspected [77].

X-rays and/or more sophisticated imaging techniques are used in imaging research. When medically prescribed conservative treatment for lower back pain fails and imaging is chosen, the examiner should begin with weight-bearing radiographs of both sides of the lumbar vertebrae (AP and lateral). If radiographs cannot explain persistent lower back pain and there is strong clinical suspicion of a systemic illness, such as red flag symptoms, advanced imaging, such as computed tomography (CT), or magnetic resonance imaging (MRI), may be useful. For the majority of patients with low back pain that require advanced imaging, an MRI without contrast is typically regarded as the best initial test [78].

Reasons for Low Back Pain

The history, physical examination, and, in rare situations, imaging of a patient can frequently help distinguish the aetiology of lower back pain. Myofascial discomfort is a frequent musculoskeletal problem, particularly following trauma or injuries from repeated activity. Facet-mediated pain is a complex process that results from intervertebral disc degeneration, which causes lumbar facet joint destruction. Facet joint osteoarthritis and tension on the facet joint's capsule can contribute to pain [79].

Discogenic pain is another typical low back pain contributor. Comer (2009) estimates that 39% of lower back pain causes are intervertebral disc-related. Internal disc rupture is primarily brought about by the disc's and its nuclear components' deterioration, however, it may also be exacerbated by the growth of radial fissures which extend from the nucleus to the annulus. Patients who are overweight or obese and consume tobacco have a greater prevalence of discogenic low back pain. Additionally, it has been discovered that patients who work physically demanding occupations that require moving heavy objects and being exposed to vibrations have a greater prevalence of illness than those who work sedentary jobs that need lengthy sitting [80].

Patients who have undergone one or more spinal operations are at risk of developing lumbar post laminectomy syndrome, often known as chronic or recurrent low back pain with or without radicular symptoms. The preoperative, intraoperative, and postoperative variables that contribute to lumbar post-laminectomy syndrome are the cause of the condition. Patients having a history of chronic anxiety, depression, or inadequate coping mechanisms are at risk before surgery. The preoperative, intraoperative, and postoperative variables that contribute to lumbar post-laminectomy syndrome are the cause of the condition. Patients having a history of chronic anxiety, depression, and inadequate coping mechanisms are at risk before surgery [81].

Pain Management For The Low Back Pain

Multidisciplinary Treatment Approach

Because not all individuals react to the same course of therapy and because no one intervention is often 100% successful for all patients, lower back pain care differs from person to person. Relevant treatment options include prescription medications, counseling, physical and occupational therapy, alternative and complementary medical techniques, or minimally invasive percutaneous techniques. Both acute and persistent lower back pain require pharmacologic therapies. It has been demonstrated that paracetamol and nonsteroidal anti-inflammatory medications (NSAIDs) are efficient for providing relief quickly. At doses up to 4 g/day, acetaminophen does not clearly differ from NSAIDs in terms of analgesia for treating acute pain. However, acetaminophen marginally falls short of NSAIDs in providing pain relief for persistent lower back pain. Both acute and persistent lower back pain require pharmacologic therapies. Short-term pain alleviation has been demonstrated to be effective with paracetamol and nonsteroidal anti-inflammatory medications (NSAIDs). At doses up to 4 g/day, acetaminophen does not clearly differ from NSAIDs in terms of analgesia for treating acute pain [82].

However, acetaminophen marginally falls short of NSAIDs in providing pain relief for persistent lower back pain. Acute and chronic low back pain are both treated with nonsteroidal anti-inflammatory medications (NSAIDs), and studies have demonstrated that both non-selective and COX-2 selective NSAIDs are more effective than placebo. It has also been demonstrated that skeletal muscle relaxants are beneficial for treating severe lower back pain. Two-week short-term studies demonstrate analgesia to be better than placebo, although there is no discernible difference between different muscle relaxants [83].

Tramadol and stronger opioids should only be used sparingly and in cases of extreme, incapacitating pain that cannot be managed by the aforementioned treatments. The analgesic effectiveness, improved activity, adverse effects, and aberrant behaviour (4A's) of these drugs should be monitored throughout their time-limited course of treatment. The usage of tricyclic antidepressants (TCA) has demonstrated positive results for the treatment of lower back pain. RCT effectiveness for persistent low back pain has been shown. TCAs work by principally inhibiting serotonin and norepinephrine reuptake, blocking sodium channels, and antagonising NMDA [84].

In addition, pharmaceutical treatments for persistent low back pain include serotonin norepinephrine reuptake inhibitors (SNRIs). Antiepileptics are also a part of pharmacologic therapy for low back pain. Only topiramate has been researched for chronic axis low back pain with evidence in analgesia and enhanced quality of life, whereas gabapentin has demonstrated analgesic effectiveness for persistent low lumbar pain with radiculopathy. Additionally, psychological therapies must be considered for application in the course for patient care because they are a crucial component of the therapy of low back pain [85].

Percutaneous approaches include manipulations on the lumbar facet (zygapophyseal) joints. Anatomical investigations have shown that the lumbar facet joints' nerve terminals are innervated by the medial branches from the dorsal rami. Intra-articular injections, medial branch nerve blocks, and radiofrequency medial branch nerve neurotomy have all been used to treat joint pain. Sacroiliac joint manipulations are yet another example of a low-risk cure for low pain in the back. Patients with spondyloarthropathies, as well as those who are older and have had post lumbar fusion, are known to experience substantial discomfort in their sacroiliac joints [86] Epidural steroid injections (ESI) are another option for treating lumbar radicular pain and spinal stenosis. The most supported RCT data for epidural steroid injections is in those who have acute radicular pain consistent with the location the lumbar disc herniation instead of axial lumbar discomfort. These individuals have considerable, albeit brief (3 month), analgesia. Last but not least, minimally invasive treatments for low back pain include spinal cord stimulation (SCS) and lumbar post-laminectomy syndrome. Epidural electrodes used in spinal cord stimulation provide electrical pulses to painful vertebral levels, either by masking the pain with paresthesia (as with classic low-frequency SCS devices) or by using high-frequency (10 kHz) non-paresthesia neuromodulation [87].

<u>Prevention of Low back Pain</u>

Lower back discomfort is primarily treated via prevention. Primal prevention, primary prevention, second- and tertiary prevention, and quaternary prevention are all different types of prevention.

Primordial prevention aims to lower risk factors across the board in order to lower the prevalence of illness. Its focus is on changing societal norms and lifestyle choices that may lead to disease. Providing sidewalks, bike lanes, open areas for leisure activities, gyms for exercise, and medical education on food, weight, alcohol, and tobacco management are fundamental preventative measures for low back pain [88].

Primary prevention focuses on lowering incidence in a group that is thought to be vulnerable to the illness, with the ultimate goal of preventing the illness from ever developing. The approaches are particular to each ailment, and the target audience is otherwise healthy people. Regarding low back pain, key preventative approaches include risk assessment, supply of lifting aids, instruction in manual handling, and provision of specialised lifting teams in susceptible groups like health professionals [89].

Secondary prevention focuses on making early diagnoses in people who initially seem to be healthy but are presenting with very early clinical features of the illness. The majority of methods are centred on screening since this technique frequently detects subclinical indicators rather than more pronounced symptoms. Secondary prevention for low back pain includes investigation and action after negative situations, such as lifting mishaps, early rehabilitation of injuries and symptoms, and presenteeism avoidance. Absenteeism is an sick absence brought on by illness. Attendance despite illness is known as presenteeism. According to certain research, presenteeism is more expensive than absenteeism [90].

Tertiary prevention focuses on lessening illness symptoms after the disease has advanced. The goal is to lessen the impact that illness has on a person's productivity and way of life. The delivery of bodily rehabilitation, cognitive behaviour therapy, and job role modifications are included in the tertiary preventive approaches for low back pain in order to prevent a recurrence [88,89]. Quaternary prevention (P4) is a concept in healthcare and medicine that focuses on actions taken to mitigate or avoid the consequences of unnecessary or excessive healthcare interventions. It is particularly relevant in situations where medical practices, including diagnosis and treatment, may do more harm than good. It extends its focus on minimizing the negative effects of medical procedures. In order to prevent low back pain, fourth prophylaxis entails avoiding surgical consequences and countless examinations in people who are anxious and also false positive cases, especially those who have an early self-limiting sickness [90].

These people require protection from actions that can produce more detrimental than beneficial results. The results of MRI scanning and several corticosteroid injections are detrimental to back pain. MRI scans may only reveal ageing-related changes and perhaps result in emotional anguish. The lack of muscular strength is the primary cause of mechanical low back pain. The foundation of muscles is destroyed by corticosteroids, which also obliterate collagen. Injecting corticosteroids into the disc gaps and facet joint is not advised [87-91]. The aforementioned interventions overlap each other quite a bit. The interventions can also be further divided into those that may be implemented by the health administration and those that can be imposed by the person.

Interventions That Can Be Set Up With The Health Facility's Administration

The purpose of this manual handling training is to teach medical professionals how to lower their risk of workplace accidents. Theis and Finkelstein demonstrated that a programme emphasising safe patient handling led to a considerable decrease in injury occurrence. They continued and came to the conclusion that for every dollar used for training, $3.71 was made [92].

A Lot Of Evidence Supports The Provision Of Lifting Equipment

Using technical equipment to help with patient handling may reduce the frequency of physical injuries within the healthcare setting.

Anyan and colleagues discovered the installation of overhead lifting systems led to a noticeably lower number of claims from medical experts as well as a lower percentage of absence and employee accidents [93].

A lift team is made up of a number of individuals who have received specialised training in lifting procedures. The lift crew rotates across the healthcare facility to assist with patient lifting throughout the day. Nursing staff embraced a lift-assist team, which reduced injuries among direct care providers; however, it is unknown if the lift assist team members have been exposed to handling risk.

A training program for healthcare personnel that aims to increase their own body awareness, improve communication with patients, and reduce injuries. It needs knowledge to instruct patients on how to take part in transfers. The educational intervention helped health workers become more adept at assisting patients in moving on their own, which served to relieve stress on both themselves and their patients [94].

A thorough ergonomic programme and patient devices reduced patient handling injuries of 59.8%, missed workdays of 86.7%, and insurance expenditures by 90.6%, according to research by Garg and colleagues.

Individual

Lifestyle Health Promotion - Although nurses are on the front lines of medical treatment, it's possible that they are unable to put the healthy living guidelines into practise. Healthy lifestyle practises are hampered by work schedules, social food customs, personnel shortages, workload, workplace stress, and shift patterns [95].

Diet - According to the government recommendations for the United Kingdom, a healthy diet should include five servings of vegetables and fruit each day. According to a survey conducted on a paediatric ward, 79% or the nurses failed to consume five servings of vegetables and fruit each day. The nurses said that promoting a nutritious diet with their patients was hindered by their absence of adherence with national norms [96].

Weight Reduction - According to a UK national survey, 25% of English doctors had a BMI above 30. Compared to other healthcare occupations, nurses had a considerably greater frequency of obesity, but unregistered carers had the highest rate [96].

Smoking - A longitudinal study conducted in seven hospitals across Italy found that a significant fraction of medical staff members smoke. Compared to other occupations, the smoking prevalence among health workers was greater [95]. The smoking rate among the 1082 healthcare professionals was 44%. Of those, 49.8% were nurses and 33.9% were doctors. 50.4% of workers were support staff, while 41.1% were technicians. However, legislative changes, medication, and behavioural treatments have improved healthcare professionals' ability to quit smoking [97].

Physical Exercise - According to Chen and colleagues, 127 nurses that had been dealing with low back pain for six months were randomly assigned to one of two groups: the experimental group. Three times each week, for 50 minutes, the experimental group engaged in stretching exercises [93]. Three times each week, the control group was told to go on with regular activities for 50 minutes. At two, four, and six months, there was statistically significant improvement on the visual analogue pain scale in the experimental group. The authors came to the conclusion that a programme of stretching exercises was an efficient and secure method of addressing low back pain among nurses [95,96].

A brief randomised control study with CBT shown that weekly pain and stress management therapy for six weeks reduced pain intensity ratings [98].

Upper Extremity Disorders

American workers frequently suffer from upper limb musculoskeletal conditions such carpal tunnel syndrome, rotator cuff tendonitis, and epicondylitis. The tissues that are impacted include blood vessels, nerves, muscles, and tendons. These conditions are more common among workers in a variety of industries, especially those that demand heavy application of the arms and hands as well as frequent exposure to vibration [95,97].

Epidemiology of Upper Extremity Disorders

Over the past 20 years, the reported prevalence of upper limb problems at work has significantly grown in the US. According to data on workplace illnesses and injuries compiled by the United States Department of Labor's Bureau of Labour Statistics (BLS), this illness category—referred to by the BLS as disorders related to repeated trauma—rose from 18% of the total number of occupational illnesses within 1982 to 65% for all occupational illnesses in 1998 [95-99]. The manufacturing of motor cars and automobile bodies, poultry slaughter and processing, clothing manufacturing, and shoe manufacturing had the greatest incidence rates for occupational illnesses linked to repetitive motion in 1998 [99]. Real estate representatives, security and commodities dealers, as well as primary and secondary school instructors, reported incredibly low incidence rates. Despite these incidence rates, the real illness burden is probably underestimated by reported work-related musculoskeletal ailments. Actual incidence rates are unclear due to underreporting by employees of their employers as well as by employers according to the Department of Labour, varied methodologies used by healthcare practitioners to determine whether an incident is work-related, and different workers' compensation laws in each state [100].On a global scale, the prevalence of upper extremity problems varies; the same is true in India. Occupational demands, lifestyle choices, and accessibility to healthcare are some of the factors that play a role. Rates could be greater in sectors that rely on physical labour, such as agriculture. Workers in offices may feel the effects of urbanisation and the rise in technological usage. The significance of customised interventions is highlighted by the fact that culturally different behaviours and a lack of awareness impact approaches to diagnosis and prevention.

Risk Factors of Upper Extremity Disorders

Occupational Risk Factors Overview

Forceful hand and arm motions, repeated hand and arm usage, actions requiring extreme hand and arm postures, extended static postures, and vibration are among the occupational risk factors that are almost widely identified as possibly contributing to upper extremity musculoskeletal diseases.

The most well-established risk factors for diseases that affect the proximal hand (tendonitis, carpal tunnel disorder, and handarm vibration syndrome) are force, repetition, and vibration.The most established risk factors for diseases of the neck and shoulder (such as trapezius myalgia and rotator cuff disorders) are posture, repetition, and force [101].

The best method of prevention is instead a "ergonomics programme" for any given workplace which involves (1) inspection for facilities for possibly dangerous exposure, (2) surveillance of staff members for unusual elevations in disease incidence, (3) monitoring of exposure when experience indicates they are likely potentially hazardous or incidence rates show an issue, (4) proper handling of clinical illness when it occurs, as well as (5) education for employees and managers [102].

Non-workplace Risk Factors

Numerous non-occupational variables also raise risk, which is true for practically all occupational diseases. Musculoskeletal diseases often occur at higher rates in women and those who are older. However, it's conceivable that these links are the result of longer exposure times and the preference given to placing women in manual labour positions. Pre-existing rheumatoid arthritis, a history of musculoskeletal disorders, and, at least for carpal tunnel syndrome, a high body mass index, pregnancy, obesity, renal dialysis, and perhaps thyroid illness, are additional risk factors [103].

Clinical assessment

A work-related musculoskeletal condition is characterised by persistent musculoskeletal discomfort or discomfort on the job. Other signs might be weakness, numbness, burning, or tingling, as well as tired muscles. Inquiring about the pain's characteristics, such as its quickness of onset, severity, quality, location, radiation, aggravating and mitigating variables, and daily patterns, might provide light on its origin. Early assessment of pain (i.e., early reporting of employees) is thought to be crucial for controlling symptoms and giving patients the chance to reduce their exposure to danger in the future [104].

Visual Inspection

Inspection, palpation, testing of passive and active ranges of motion, assessment of nervous system health, and pulse checking should all be included in a physical examination. There are several great manuals for physical examinations of the upper extremities.

Laboratory Assessment

Laboratory testing are primarily used to exclude systemic disease as the primary cause and contributor to musculoskeletal complaints. An infection, osteoarthritis, gout, calcium pyrophosphate depositing, diabetes, hypothyroidism, and collagen vascular disease are examples of systemic illnesses. The choice of further tests, including electromyography, radiologic imaging, and nerve conduction testing, is also based in the differential diagnosis made after the assessment. However, unless an underlying disease is detected, laboratory testing is typically not necessary during the time the initial examination [105].

The majority of occupational musculoskeletal diseases should start with conservative treatments such rest, anti-inflammatory drugs, cold and heat packs, and physical or occupational therapy. Controlling exposures that contributed to the onset of occupational musculoskeletal illnesses is essential to their treatment. Treatment that doesn't address the workplace issues that contributed to the problem is likely to fail. Transferring the worker to another position, limiting the amount of time the worker is exposed to his regular work activities (restricted duty), redesigning the workspace and tasks, changing work procedures like rotating the workforce and increasing rest breaks, and using personal protective equipment are all examples of exposure control. Rarely, and only after conservative treatment has failed, can surgery be considered for occupational musculoskeletal diseases [106].

Short Shoulder Disorders

The shoulder has a wide range of movement and is prone to harm at work.% It can be challenging to classify shoulder diseases, especially when the symptoms are severe and persistent.

Truncal myalgia

Localised pain in the trapezius muscles is referred to as trapezius myalgia. It is also known as tension head syndrome on occasion. The majority of working populations are affected by this illness, which is the most prevalent among occupational shoulder and neck ailments [107].

Therapeutic Presentation:

Patients typically complain of the upper back, shoulder, and regions immediately lateral to the neck discomfort, tightness, stiffness, or burning. Physical examination may reveal muscular tension and "trigger points" of heightened muscle tone and discomfort. There might be slight reductions in the range of motion.

Risk Elements:

Data entering on a computer terminal is an example of a job duty that requires constant neck, shoulder, and back posture. Unchanging immobile posture of the neck, shoulder, and back as well as extended static stress of the shoulder muscles are occupational risk factors. People who work in assembly line manufacturing, dentistry, some medical specialties, fine electrical or microelectronics, artisanal or jewelry-making, or office jobs like data entry or keyboarding are all susceptible to this condition [108].

Treatment:

Applications of heat and ice may help with symptoms. Low dosages of tricyclic antidepressants can prove helpful for the management of pain and enhancement of sleep in patients with severely incapacitating symptoms. At the very least, continuing vigorous usage of the shoulders and arms won't hurt, and it could even help with symptoms.

Tendonitis of the rotator cuff

The tendons that make up the rotator cuff (Figure 12) are affected by rotator cuff tendonitis, sometimes referred to as supraspinatus tendonitis. The functional unit made from the supraspinatus, infraspinatus, and subscapularis muscles is known as the rotator cuff. The impingement of rotator cuff structures on the bone underneath them results in tendonitis of the shoulder, as shown in Figure 13 [109].

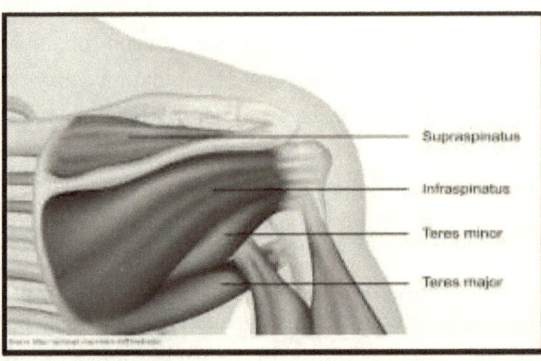

Figure 12: Muscles attached with the posterior aspect of the spine

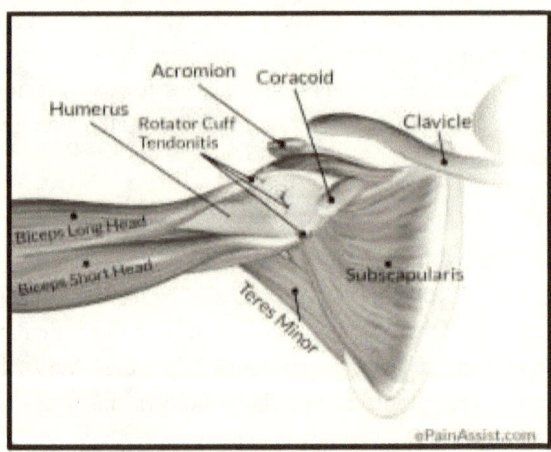

Figure 13: Rotator cuff tendonitis

Therapeutic Presentation:

Although it may spread down the arm, discomfort often localises in the superior and lateral shoulder in clinical terms. When the arc-of-motion test is affirmative, The Huwkins' impingement sign, or forward flexion of a shoulder to 90 degrees with internal rotation on the humerus, repeats The afflicted arm's muscle may be healthy or somewhat weaker.

Risk Elements:

The risk of rotator cuff tendonitis increases when a worker does forceful or repeated tasks involving any movement of the shoulder, but especially abduction, flexion, and rotation. Rotator cuff tendinitis is more likely to develop as a result of overhead labour, such as holding a tool with one hand or above shoulder height, as well as vigorous activities involving frequent tugging or lifting.IBt38 The likelihood of developing shoulder tendonitis may also be increased by strenuous lifting and immobile upper body positions. Plumbing, mechanical maintenance, construction, factory and manufacturing work, poultry machines, riveters, welders, mail transporters, telephone managers, grocery store checkers, for instance, garment manufacturers, orchard workers, as well as dentists are a few examples of occupations at risk [110].

Treatment:

In order to prevent the side effects of adhesive capsulitis and frozen shoulder syndrome, conservative therapy calls for resting the shoulder but not immobilising it. This can entail limiting arm lifting and refraining from any overhead work for one to three weeks. Anti-inflammatory drugs alleviate symptoms. Steroidal injections decrease acute pain, but because of how slowly they work, they should only be used in certain circumstances.

After initial symptoms have subsided, physical therapy should start, progressing from modest range-of-motion activities to strengthening ones. When conservative approaches are ineffective, surgery may be considered [111].

Bursitis of the subdelta

An inflammatory condition of the subdeltoid bursa is known as subdeltoid bursitis. The subdeltoid bursa constitutes a sac the size of a palm that is located below the rotator cuff and below the deltoid muscle. Subacromial bursitis is another name for subdeltoid bursitis because the deltoid bursa spreads below the bone acromion.

Therapeutic Presentation:

The majority of the symptoms include dull, throbbing discomfort, swelling, and limited shoulder motion. The signs and symptoms may be difficult to distinguish from rotator cuff tendinitis. The discomfort may worsen at night and manifest as shoulder pressure when lying flat. On physical examination, the deltoid area could feel painful. Pain may make it difficult to do a shoulder abduction as well as a forward flexion physical examination. Muscle power ought to be unaffected. Comparison of the injured shoulder with the contralateral shoulder is necessary [112].

Risk Elements:

Repetitive use of one's upper extremities with shoulder motion, especially overhead labour, is a risk factor for subdeltoid bursitis. Changing the workday routine is one method of prevention that aims to lessen shoulder activity. Subdeltoid bursitis may be avoided by reducing mechanical pressures on the shoulder via modifications to workplace layout and the adoption of lighter items and supplies.

Treatment:

Resting the shoulder is part of the treatment. Applications of cold, heat, and anti-inflammatory medications lessen discomfort. When initial symptoms lessen, physical treatment for light reconditioning is advised. In situations that are severe or chronic, corticosteroid injections into the bursa may be able to offer relief.

Bifid Tendonitis

Inflammation on the biceps tendon and tendon sheath within the bicipital groove on the more anterior proximal humerus is known as bicipital tendonitis.

Therapeutic Presentation:

Anterior shoulder discomfort and soreness are signs of bicipital tendonitis. Biceps tendon probing at the front shoulder always reveals considerable soreness. Resisting flexion of the shoulder while keeping the elbow extended completely and the forearm supinated also causes pain [113].

Risk Elements:

Asking people who have biceps tendon discomfort about aggravating work-related motions, such as direct damage to the tendon, and leisure activities, such as playing sports, is important. Risk factors include persistent shoulder postures, particularly in flexion and abduction, as well as highly repetitive jobs requiring shoulder movement. Heavy equipment assembly, red meat abattoir labour, agricultural work or harvesting, production, manufacturing work, and food store checking are among the occupations linked to bicipital tendonitis.

Treatment:

Anti-inflammatory drugs, and cold, and heat treatments are used as conservative treatment methods. Resting the arm and biceps is advised. Physical therapy may assist with progressive biceps restrengthening when acute symptoms have subsided. Although they sometimes result in relief, local injections of steroids into the bicipital tendon raise the risk of tendon rupture [114].

Disorders of the elbow Lateral Epicondylitis

A condition of pain in the wrist extensor muscles located near or around its lateral epicondyle origin and discomfort right over the epicondyle is known as lateral epicondylitis, often known as tennis elbow.

Clinical traits:

The patient often complains of elbow pain on the lateral side. On physical examination, the proximal extensor muscles or point discomfort at or just distal to the lateral epicondyle are both evident.

Risk Elements:

Forearm rotation that is repeated, such as when using a screwdriver, has been linked by some researchers to lateral epicondylitis. Another symptom of this disease is a strong grasp with an extended wrist [115].

Treatment:

The condition could only slowly get better. Rest, splinting, cold and heat treatments, as well as anti-inflammatory or pain drugs, are all forms of therapy.

Exercises for stretching and strengthening are advised when acute symptoms have subsided. Modifying work processes and equipment is a part of prevention. The execution of job activities while the palm up can change labour motions, reducing dependence upon the lateral flexor muscles [116].

Epicondylitis in the media

A condition known as "golfer's elbow" or medial epicondylitis causes discomfort in the wrist flexor and extensor muscles close to the origin of those muscles, or immediately above the epicondyle.

Clinical traits:

The medial epicondyle is sensitive upon physical examination.

The medial elbow hurts when the wrist is flexed against resistance.

Risk Elements:

The existence of medial epicondylitis as an occupational condition is not well established.

Treatment:

To protect the wounded epicondyle when resting on its side on hard surfaces, elbow protectors are advised. Limiting exposure could promote healing. While there are other treatments that are comparable to those for lateral epicondylitis, steroid injection is not advised [115,117].

Disorders of the Distal Upper Extremity

DeQuervain's Syndrome

Stenosing tenosynovitis of the thumb's extensor tendons is referred to as DeQuervain's disease when it causes discomfort across the radial styloid process and impairs thumb function.

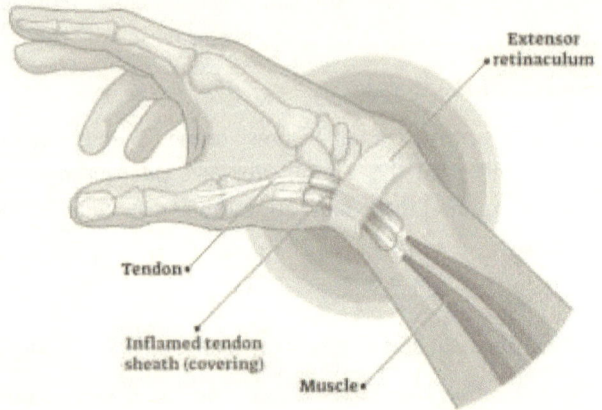

Figure 14: Inflammation in the tendon sheath and thumb's extensor tendons, referred to as DeQuervain's disease

Clinical traits:

Pain, potential edema, and heat of the radial wrist are symptoms. The thumb's abduction and extension make the discomfort greater [118]. Physical examination may indicate nodules, soreness, and discomfort along the wrist's radial artery.

Risk Elements:

Assembly line work, the creation of tiny items, the processing of meat and poultry, the manufacturing of textiles, the packaging of food, the use of computers and keypunching have all been linked to DeQuervain's illness. DeQuervain's illness has been linked to repeated hand motions, frequent thumb extension, and significant lateral wrist deviations in the workplace.

Treatment:

Anti-inflammatory drugs, rest using the thumb inside a spica splint, and occupational or physical therapy are all part of the treatment. A study of conservative therapy can be followed with cortisone injections [119].

Forearm and wrist flexor tendonitis

Forearm extensor tendon pain is a symptom of tendonitis of the forearm and wrist extensors. There are several diagnostic entities, and any of the wrist's dorsal compartments might be impacted.

Extensor indicis and extensor carpi ulnaris tendinitis are two examples.

Clinical traits:

Tenderness, swelling, warmth, irritation, or crepitance may accompany pain. All symptoms should be able to be pinpointed to specific extensor compartments or areas that lie on the dorsum of one's hand, wrist, or forearm [120].

Risk Elements:

The risk for extensor tendonitis is increased by repetitive, strong hand use, using the hands at the limits of their joint range of motion, and doing strange or unfamiliar activities.

Treatment:

The first stage of clinical therapy consists of nonsteroidal anti-inflammatory drugs, rest, and splinting. The effectiveness of physical and occupational therapy may vary. Only refractory patients should receive steroid injections.

Forearm and wrist flexor tendonitis

When volar forearm discomfort is brought on by resisted wrist and digital flexion, tendonitis affecting the forearm and wrist flexors is suspected [121].

Clinical traits:

Physical examination may reveal redness, swelling, warmth, or (occasionally) crepitus in addition to tenderness to palpation. An important diagnostic symptom is pain with resisted bending of the hand and fingers. Alternative sources of pain should be examined, such as median or ulnar neuropathies.

Risk Elements:

Similar to extensor tendonitis, flexor tendonitis is more likely to develop in those who use their hands repeatedly, forcefully, or at extremes of their joint range of motion [122].

Tensor tendonitis treatment

The same procedure is used to treat wrist flexor tendonitis and trigger finger. In order to impede smooth tendon movement, the trigger finger is brought about by swelling in the finger flexor tendon and constriction of the tendons pulley superficial of the middle metacarpal (MCP) joint.

clinical traits:

The symptoms of the trigger finger include locking or triggering of the fingers and soreness or crepitance within the wrist flexor tendon sheath near the A1 pulley. Due to locking in flexion and extension, the afflicted finger may have a reduced range of motion. A defining characteristic of the condition is pain that may be palpated immediately above the MCP joint [123].

Risk Elements:

There isn't much evidence linking a job to having a trigger finger. The region has likely been subjected to frequent renovation and pressure from hard items, such as tool handles.

Treatments:

The preferred therapies include steroid injections, nonsteroidal anti-inflammatory drugs, and bracing. It has been said that surgically releasing the fibrotic tendon is effective [124].

Neck And Cervical Spine Disorders

The International Association for Ergonomics (IEA) defines ergonomics as the scientific field that studies how people interact with other system components [121]. The science of ergonomics focuses on making a worker's workspace efficient, safe, secure, and enjoyable so that they enjoy producing valuable outputs for the business they work for. Today's excessive use of electronics and mobile devices raises the danger of a variety of musculoskeletal issues, which ought to be taken seriously [122]. Numerous researchers claim that prolonged usage of these gadgets results in bad posture and an elevated risk of injury. According to several studies, working more than 5 hours while seated at a desk and sleeping seven hours at night have a major negative influence on mental and physical well-being [123-125].

Another approach is to use therapeutic exercises to correct any muscular imbalances that could be a factor in the motion compensation that causes neck pain [124]. Deep cervical flexor exercises and retraining are employed in clinical settings to relieve neck discomfort and improve the ability to maintain a standing position [125]. Therapeutic activities are advised in neck pain therapy for individuals with chronic neck pain, poor posture, along with other health conditions due to their major influence. Resistance training and endurance training decreased pain and impairment ratings in office employees with chronic neck discomfort, according to O'Riordan et al. (2014) [126].

Training in Ergonomics

For the avoidance of work-related upper-limb and neck musculoskeletal diseases, ergonomic counsel suggests ergonomic training when using a desktop computer. Avoid performing repetitive jobs since they could make you feel more exhausted [125,126]. A very low or high workstation might also make it difficult for one's upper extremity to retain it in place for extended periods of time, leading to muscle exhaustion. Forearms and hands should be roughly horizontal with the chair for comfort. The elbows ought to be placed vertically behind the shoulder when placing the fingers on the middle row of the keyboard to avoid creating an angle in the wrist joint. The feet ought to be level with the ground. It is necessary to blink regularly every two hours [127].

Glare reducing screen filters can be utilised for the optimal illumination. If the chair isn't comfortable, lumbar pillows might be employed. ergonomically designed. Avoid adopting an unpleasant sitting position, and switch positions often. Making frequent should become ingrained with you [126,127]. Avoid placing the screen too near to the eyes as this might lead to neither can it be too far on one side since this puts a disproportionate amount of strain upon the eyes, which might cause vision-related issues in throat muscles. When working, both hands ought to be utilised symmetrically. Using a chair that has a footrest guarantee. so the pressure is evenly distributed and eased from the thigh [128].

A document holder may be set up on top of the desk to lessen neck and spinal strain at work. It needs to be situated at the same level and distance from the monitor. All of the workplace accoutrements, including phones, paper trays, and bottles, should be easily reachable. When possible, try to avoid reaching and twisting [129].

Therapeutic Exercises And Ergonomic Training

Another approach is to use therapeutic exercises to correct any muscular imbalances that could be a factor in the movement compensating that causes neck pain. Deep cervical flexor exercises and retraining are employed in clinical settings to relieve neck discomfort and improve the ability to maintain a standing position [130]. Therapeutic activities are recommended for neck pain treatment in those with chronic cervical pain, poor posture, and additional health conditions since they have such a big influence. The secret to effectively retraining therapeutic exercise effectiveness over the long run may be to maintain great posture when exercising. When it came to neck discomfort and poor posture, ergonomic training and therapeutic exercises worked best [131].

Neck pain

Neck pain is a type of discomfort that originates in the neck and may radiate down either one or both arms. Numerous conditions or illnesses that affect the neck's tissues, nerves, bones, joints, ligaments, or muscles can cause neck discomfort. The cervical spine, or neck part of the spinal column, is made from 7 bones (C1-C7 vertebrae), that are spaced apart by intervertebral discs. These discs provide the spine with mobility and serve as shock absorbers while people are moving about.

The entire length of the back is made up of a single hollow longitudinal space formed by openings in each vertebral bone. The vertebral column and nerve bundles flow through this location, known as the spinal canal. The dura, a leathery sac-like layer of protection, surrounds the spinal cord and is encased in the cerebrospinal fluid (CSF) that surrounds it [132].

Two sets of spinal nerves emerge from each level of the vertebra through two tiny holes called foramina, one on the left and another to the right. All regions of the body experience sensation and movement thanks to the delivery of these nerves to the muscles, skin, and other bodily tissues. The fragile spinal cord and nerves are shielded by the bone vertebrae and suspended by the spinal fluid within the dural sac. Strong muscles and ligaments that bind and provide safe movement further support the bony vertebrae [130-132].

Causes

Arthritis, disc degeneration, spinal canal constriction, muscular inflammation, strain, or trauma can all lead to neck discomfort. Rarely, it could be a symptom of meningitis or malignancy. For proper diagnosis and treatment recommendations for major neck issues, an ordinary doctor should be contacted as well as frequently a specialist, like a neurosurgeon [133].

Age, trauma, bad posture, or illnesses like arthritis can cause the cervical spine's bones or joints to degenerate, which can result in disc herniation or the formation of bone spurs. Sudden, severe neck injuries can cause discs herniation, whiplash, damage to blood vessels, spinal injury, and in the worst cases, they can cause lifelong paralysis. The spinal canal, or the tiny apertures through which the spinal nerve roots exit, may become narrowed by herniated discs and bone spurs, placing pressure on the spinal cord and the nerves [134].

Since almost all of the nerves that travel to the remainder of the body (arms, chest, abdomen, and legs) must pass through the neck in order to reach their destination, tension on the spinal cord within the cervical area can be a major issue. Numerous crucial organs' ability to operate may be jeopardised by this. Numbness, discomfort, or weakness in the arm region that the nerve feeds can occur when a nerve is under pressure [135].

Injuries

Neck stiffness, discomfort in the shoulder or arm, headache, pain in the face, and vertigo are all signs of a neck injury. Tears in the muscles or damage of the joints between the vertebrae may result in pain after a motor vehicle accident. Damage to a spinal disc or a ruptured ligament are additional sources of discomfort. Medication for the discomfort, a decrease in physical activity, and physical therapy are all considered conservative treatments for these ailments [136].

Symptoms

With addition to neck discomfort, a herniated disc and a bone spur pressing upon a nerve root and the spinal cord may cause:

- There is arm pain.
- Arm or forearm numbness or a feeling of weakness
- Tingle in the hands or fingers
- difficulty walking and balancing
- The legs or arms are weakened

Cervical spine disorders

The majority of individuals who complain of neck discomfort have "nonspecific (simple) neck pain," in which the cause is mechanical or postural. Aetiological variables, such as incorrect posture, depressive disorders, anxiety, neck strain, and sports or occupational activities, are typically complex and poorly understood. If there is no bone damage or neurological impairment, neck pain following a whiplash injury also falls under this group [137].

The term "cervical spondylosis," although it is frequently used to refer to any non-specific neck pain, is frequently used when mechanical reasons are prevalent in the disorder.

Chronic neck discomfort is more likely to have mechanical and generative causes.

In cervical spondylosis, osteophyte production and involvement of nearby soft tissue structures are the first signs of degenerative alterations in the intervertebral discs.

On simple radiographs showing the cervical spine, many persons over 30 have comparable anomalies, making it challenging to distinguish between normal aging and illness. Although severe degenerative changes are frequently asymptomatic, they might cause neurological issues, neck discomfort, or stiffness [138].

Anyone who has neck pain?

Neck discomfort affects over two thirds of people at some point in their life, and frequency is highest in middle age. 25% of women and 20% of men in a general practise survey of persons in the United Kingdom reported having neck discomfort right now. In a poll of 10,000 individuals conducted in Norway, 34% of participants reported having neck discomfort in the year prior. Neck discomfort is the second most common musculoskeletal reason for primary care consultations globally, after back pain. About 15% of hospital-based physiotherapy in the UK and 30% of chiropractic recommendations in Canada are made due to neck discomfort [139].

Neck pain epidemiological studies frequently rely on questionnaires or demographic surveys and may overstate the condition's prevalence. Despite these methodological challenges, they do show that neck discomfort has a significant negative impact on people, companies, and healthcare systems.

What are the typical causes of neck pain?

The result of neck pain depends upon the underlying cause, although acute neck pain often goes away within a few days or weeks unless it recurs or develops into chronic neck pain (lasting more than three months). Once pain becomes chronic, the outcome is unknown, and the prognosis and the variables affecting it vary widely. There are different reports about the significance of variables including age, sex, employment, psychological issues, and radiological results, however, the majority of research quality is subpar [140].

More than 10% of those who are impacted experience persistent neck discomfort, while other studies indicate that this number is far higher. In certain professions, neck-related illnesses cause as much time away from work as low back discomfort. In 5% of sufferers, neck discomfort results in severe impairment.

How is cervical spine degeneration identified?

Although discomfort is often within the area of the cervical spine, it may relate to a wide range of locations and is frequently made worse by neck movement. When cervical spondylosis (Table 10) becomes complicated by myelopathy and radiculopathy, as well as when unconnected causes like disc prolapse, thoracic connection obstruction, brachial plexus disease, malignancy, and primary neurological disease are present, it is always important to look for neurological change in the upper and lower limbs. However, objective changes only happen in these situations [141].

Table 10: Clinical Features of cervical spondylosis

Signs and Symptoms	Clinical Characteristics
Symptoms of cervical spondylosis	Ø Movement-aggravated cervical pain Ø Referred pain in the upper body (occiput, shoulder blades, limbs) Ø (C1 to C2) Temporal or retro-orbital discomfort Ø Reversible or irreversible cervical stiffness Ø Upper limb weakness, tingling, or generalised numbness Ø nausea or vertigo Ø bad balance Ø Occasionally, syncope, migraines, and "pseudo-angina"
Signs of cervical spondylosis	Ø Poor localization of tenderness Ø restricted range of motion (lateral flexion, forward flexion, backward extension, and rotation to both sides) Ø Minor neurological alterations, such as inverted supinator jerks (unless myelopathy or radiculopathy complicates the situation)

Epidemiology

The second most common cause of musculoskeletal diseases is neck discomfort brought on by different cervical spine abnormalities. With a rate of 83.1 per 100,000 people in the US. Both the general public and those receiving workers' compensation frequently experience neck discomfort. Over the course of a year, the prevalence of neck discomfort varies from 1.7% to 11.5% worldwide. The majority of cases occur between the years of 50 and 54, with the average age of onset being between 40 and 60.4,5 Additionally, women experience it more frequently than males do, as do metropolitan areas as opposed to rural ones, and higher-income nations as opposed to lower-income nations [142].

In asymptomatic individuals above the age of 40 and 80% of patients over the age of 80, cervical spondylosis—also known as evidence of arthritic changes—has been identified in 60% of cases. Rarely do we observe these cervical abnormalities in young children. Osteoarthritis, cervical strains, and past neck injuries all raise a patient's likelihood of developing neck discomfort [143].

Therapeutic presentations

Cervical disc disease: Cervical spondylosis, sometimes referred to as degeneration, is the most prevalent condition affecting the cervical spine. A normal element of aging is the degeneration of cervical discs. The segments from C4 to C5, C5 to C6, and C6 to C7 are the ones that are most affected by the degree of extension and flexion of the spine on these levels. Osteophytic spurring, facet joint enlargement, posterior longitudinal ligament calcification, and *ligamentum flavum* thickening are other degenerative alterations [144].

These arthritic alterations can cause tightness and stiffness within the motion segments, which in turn causes the cervical spine's natural lordosis to disappear. Mechanical in nature, spondylosis pain is characterised as a deep, slow throbbing aching with sporadic stiffness and/or headaches [142,143]. The pain usually originates posteriorly across the midline and paraspinal aspects, although it can also radiate to the shoulders via the dermatome, occiput, trapezii, and scapulae. Herniated cervical disc. This disease, which is often located over the lower segments between C4 to C7, is linked to mechanical stress, these can result in osteophytes, inflammation, bulging disc material, and/or facet joint degeneration, each of which can result in nerve impingement [144]. However, trauma may result in herniation, which is often brought on by compressive or hyperflexion forces. In 80% of instances, disc herniation symptoms are comparable to those of spondylosis, but they typically feature radiating neuropathic pain known as cervical radiculopathy [145].

Numbness, tingling, combustion, shooting, stabbing, as well as electrical shocks throughout the upper part of the body (unilateral or bilateral) are common descriptions of cervical radicular discomfort. The dermatomal pattern of these aches has the potential to cause sensory, motor, and reflex impairments. Additionally, the discomfort may go across, between, or in some cases within an anterior cape arrangement between the scapulae and clavicles. Turning and bending the head in the opposite direction from the cause usually makes the pain worse. Many patients claim that placing their ipsilateral arm over the top of their head—the abduction relief sign—or turning their head in the opposite direction reduces their pain [146].

Vertebral stenosis: Narrowing the neural foraminal, medial recesses, or central canal is known as cervical stenosis [142]. It may be classified as either congenital, which is linked to an abnormal spinal canal development that causes spinal canal constriction independent of degenerative alterations, or as degenerative, which is related to disc degeneration, aspect hypertrophy, kyphosis, or ligamentum flavum hypertrophy. In addition to the spondylosis symptoms discussed before, stenosis symptoms can also include radiculopathy. Patients who are older than 50 years old frequently develop stenosis [144-147].

Myelopathy of the neck: Long-term compression on the spinal cord can cause a condition called cervical myelopathy, which is incurable if left untreated. It usually starts slowly and progresses step by step, with intervals of static function. Worldwide, cervical myelopathy is the most common cause of age spinal cord dysfunction and is mainly encountered in those over the age of 55. The development of fine motor problems, such as grip difficulty, the inability to operate buttons or zippers, imbalance, gait disturbances, changes in sensory function, hyperreflexia, abnormal, spasms, and bladder or bowel incontinence, are typical symptoms that usually follow the dermatomal pattern of the present vertebral level [148].

Stability of the spinal column: The rigidity of the spinal column is impacted by a number of different conditions. The majority of spinal column instability is caused by both degenerative and traumatic influences. Spondylolisthesis, which is frequently caused by disc or facet degeneration, is the anterior and posterior spinal displacement to the next vertebra. Due to muscular stiffness, cervical sprains might show loss of lordosis, which is the cervical spine's natural curvature. The reversal of lordosis, known as kyphosis, is linked to severe spondylosis or trauma [147,149].

Fractures: Fractures can happen at any level of the vertebrae and are frequently brought on by trauma to the spine. The term "Jefferson fracture" refers to an atlas (C1) fracture. A hangman's fracture is a traumatic spondylolisthesis that affects the cervical axis (C2), whereas an odontoid fracture, classified as Type I to III based on the site, is a fracture of the C2 body [147,148]. Every vertebral body can have compression fractures due to trauma or pathological conditions like multiple myeloma. With or without instability, fractures can also develop along the facet joint itself. Rarely do transverse or spinous process fractures lead to instability [149].

Examining a patient with neck pain

If a patient has neck discomfort, you should first evaluate whether the causes are primarily mechanical or neuropathic. It is also important to categorise neck discomfort according to how long it lasts, including acute pain lasting a maximum of six weeks, subacute pain lasting between six weeks and three months, and chronic pain lasting more than three months. A thorough physical and medical history are the best methods for establishing this conclusion [150].

The patient's history should be detailed and include the mechanism of the injury, the location of the pain and whether it reflects the shoulder and scapulae, whether there is unilateral or bilateral arm pain, balance, and gait issues, pain with lateral, flexion, and/or extension ranges of motion, sensorimotor deficits, and aggravating or mitigating factors. Keep records of previous successful or unsuccessful therapies, particularly how you responded to certain drug regimens [148-150]. A complete physical examination should include checking the spine for alignment, discomfort, and any erythema or edema, analysing the gait pattern, testing motor function for weakness, evaluating the sensory function for dermatomal abnormalities, and testing reflexes [149,151].

A Hoffman sign is normally symptomatic of a lesion of the upper motor neuron although can occasionally be a false-positive finding for some individuals. It is evoked by the downward flicking of the middle fingernail and is deemed positive with the flicking of the thumb, index, and ring finger. When a patient complains of bladder or bowel incontinence, a rectal examination is required [150-152]. In addition to the Lhermitte sign, additional provocative procedures such as the Spurling, shoulder abduction, and upper limb tension tests are employed to detect radiculopathy or cord compression. The Spurling test includes gently applying downward axial compression while rotating the patient's head in opposite and ipsilateral directions to the discomfort. A favourable outcome reproduces radicular discomfort brought on by neural foramen constriction [152].

As previously mentioned, shoulder abduction is a sign of radicular symptoms. Due to its high sensitivity and low specificity, the upper limb tension test is not as commonly employed to rule out radiculopathy [150-152]. The Lhermitte sign refers to an electrical feeling that occurs when a patient flexes and extends their head. It can also occur in the arms and/or legs. Although the sensitivity of the Lhermitte sign is less than 20%, it can indicate cord compression [153].

Diagnostic assessment of a patient with neck pain

Clinical recommendations state that routine imaging, particularly plain radiographs, was not necessary owing to radiation exposure and pathology detection, which is not always treatable. Plain anterior/posterior and lateral radiographs can be done without the addition with flexion/extension images if there's a concern for spinal instability, red flags, a history of trauma, and the patient has failed conservative therapies after 6 weeks. Employ an MRI to evaluate all cervical spinal disorders in individuals who have ongoing or developing neurologic involvement. For patients who cannot have an MRI, this is followed with a CT scan (computed tomography) and a CT myelogram, with the latter being preferred if there is a possibility of neurologic impingement. Only individuals who have already had surgery are in need of contrast MRI or CT. The existence of a hyperintense region close to the spondylotic spine is a significant T2-weighted MRI finding for individuals with cervical myelopathy [154].

Diagnosis and differentials

Any cervical spine abnormalities must be ruled up before serious pathology is identified. This includes pain that doesn't go away in any position, that gets worse at night or while you're sleeping, that's linked to trauma, an infection, a cancer, severe neurologic symptoms, or that affects people who are younger than 20 or older than 50. An electromyography and/or a nerve conduction test can help to clarify and perhaps diagnose ulnar neuropathy or carpal tunnel syndrome in individuals who have more distal than proximal peripheral neuropathy and whose radicular symptoms differ from MRI findings. Brown-Séquard syndrome, Guillain-Barré syndrome, brachial plexus injuries, and thoracic outlet syndrome are some further potential diagnoses with neurologic abnormalities in the upper extremities. Atlantoaxial and subaxial subluxation can result from rheumatoid arthritis. Marfan syndrome, a form of widespread idiopathic skeletal hyperostosis, and ossification of the posterior transverse ligament are further inflammatory and spondylotic disorders that affect the spine [155].

Neck movement limitations and discomfort can result from congenital malformations such as Klippel-Feil syndrome. Postoperatively, adjacent segment degeneration, or the degeneration of a disc located above or below a recently fused disc, might take place. Cervical spondylosis has been shown to occur four times more frequently in those with metabolic syndrome [156].

Management of Neck Pain

Cohort studies have shown a connection between longer pain duration and a worse outcome. The majority of people with acute neck discomfort will have relief in 2 months. Even cervical radiculopathy or stenosis symptoms may resolve spontaneously in 40% to 76% of cases over a varied period of time without medical intervention or surgery. To attain the results of pain alleviation, increased function, and improved quality of life, some patients will need aid through conservative therapies, which should always be the first choice in the absence of a major disease. However, the overall strength of the evidence for any intervention is still weak [157].

Nonpharmacologic: Electrical nerve stimulation through the skin (TENS), ultrasonography, acupuncture, physiotherapy, cervical traction, abuse, and electrical nerve stimulation through the skin are some of the conventional nonpharmacologic therapies for cervical spine diseases. Randomised controlled trials have demonstrated that physical therapy can alleviate acute neck pain but that independent home exercise programmes, which are supported by low-quality data from Cochrane Reviews, are ineffective in managing chronic pain. According to Cochrane Review data, traction did not work for people with chronic neck pain, however, it did in certain cases for those with acute neck pain. Additionally, manipulation showed weak support from a comprehensive review for usage in treating acute neck pain, was unsupported for treating chronic pain, and care was advised due to the possibility of symptom worsening, particularly in cervical myelopathy patients. TENS was determined by the Cochrane Review to be more beneficial than a placebo, whereas ultrasound therapy for neck pain was not supported by any research. Systematic research did establish the benefits of acupuncture for temporary pain alleviation. In summary, the majority of research found that using multimodality techniques was more successful than using single modality therapies [158].

Pharmacologic: According to the Cochrane Review and other systematic studies, there is insufficient evidence to support drug treatment, particularly when taking into account side effects. Due to its low risk of adverse effects, paracetamol has been suggested as first-line treatment when utilising drugs, however, it should be avoided in individuals with severe hypovolemia, severe renal impairment, or hepatic contraindications. Nonsteroidal anti-inflammatory drugs (NSAIDs) may be used by healthcare professionals to treat neck pain, but they come with a boxed warning for gastrointestinal (GI) along with cardiovascular (CV) side effects and should not be used in patients in GI bleeding history or those who are at high risk for bleeding, as well as those who have CV disease or CV risk factors. The use of NSAIDs carries the risk of hepatotoxicity and renal toxicity as well. Using muscle relaxants to relieve acute pain is more successful than managing chronic pain. Because of their propensity for abuse and lack of increased effectiveness, benzodiazepines are not advised. opiate analgesics should only be used in patients with intractable pain that has not responded to previous therapies, for a brief period of time, and only as a supplement to other conservative therapy methods. Patients should also be closely monitored by healthcare professionals for opiate abuse [159].

Injection treatment: Limited high-quality studies within systematic reviews acknowledged the use of cervical transforaminal epidural injections of corticosteroid as a mainstay in the treatment of cervical radiculopathy to be used after failing at least 6 weeks of alternate conservative management. There is little support for alternative injections, such as radiofrequency ablation, medial branch nerve injections, or trigger point injections in myofascial pain. Selective nerve core blocks, which are frequently used as diagnostic injections, showed a link with successful surgical results in patients who responded well. Injection-related problems can range in severity from mild ones like bleeding to more significant ones like spinal cord as well nerve injuries, epidural hematomas, or infection [160].

Surgery: Surgery is often advised as the primary choice for managing cervical myelopathy if a patient's pain does not improve with conservative therapy and they show signs of neurologic involvement, and this is according to systematic reviews. Depending on the condition, surgeries are often carried out using either anterior or posterior methods. The conventional technique for single- to triple-level disc herniation with radiculopathy / myelopathy involves anterior cervical decompression and fusion (ACDF). Patients that underwent an ACDF along with physiotherapy had better results than those who had simply received physiotherapy, according to a randomised research lasting 5 to 8 years. Posterior procedures are more frequently employed for multilayer stenosis, myelopathy, or poor surgical results. It is very advised that patients stop smoking before having surgery [161].

Patient education and prevention measures

The evaluation and treatment of psychological risk factors, or "yellow flags," which might impede rehabilitation, result in an onset of chronic pain, or result in long-term impairment, is the most crucial therapeutic approach for cervical spine problems. Socioeconomic reasons, decreased activity levels, the status of compensation or legal claims, perceptions that spinal pain is extremely incapacitating, and demands for opioid drugs when they are not appropriate for therapy are a few examples. Education on the diagnosis, which encourages self-management, reassurance, and support for maintaining an active lifestyle, should come first in all patient treatments. To help manage psychosocial risk factors, cognitive behavioural therapy is a viable and affordable approach. Collaboration in decision-making, particularly when it comes to decisions on treatment plans, including surgery, is another helpful tool for the management of neck pain [162].

Neck exercises and postural corrections

Programmes with daily exercise during a 10-week period had positive benefits on neck pain reduction and isometric strength development. Despite the fact that the study indicated a workout

Frequency:

Adherence to an exercise routine seems to vary quite a bit depending on design (e.g., three times per week). Despite the fact that people exercised on average three times per week, multiple studies, including one by Viljanen et al., indicated that over the course of twelve weeks of training adherence seldom exceeded about 39% (1.7 times/week) above anticipated statistics [163].

Intensity:

Depending on whether resistance or endurance exercise was being studied, training intensity differed. Exercises in resistance programmes are often based on percentages between 20% to 70% of a person's maximum voluntary contraction (MVC). Initial measurements of MVC were taken for strength or resistance training utilising manual muscle testing techniques with portable dynamometers or specially made fixed-frame dynamometers, or it is typically observed, repeated, or 12 repetition maximums. The capacity of a bigger set of muscles to enhance muscular stamina during endurance training, such as deep or superficial cervical muscles and greater shoulder muscles, can have an impact. circulatory system to provide blood enriched with oxygen to the region being worked out. These therapies, which focused mostly on gravity and were of lower intensity, aimed to improve physical muscle endurance. Low-dose or low-load endurance exercise programmes were still observed to have positive effects, despite the fact that high-dose/intensity exercise programmes were seen to reduce neck discomfort. Gravity was used to determine the severity of the treatments for endurance, such as supine resting and elevating the head against gravity [164].

Time:

The duration of the intervention and the amount of time that participants spent doing physical activity in a single session ranged between Due to participant non-adherence after an initial supervised exercise intervention has finished, it is challenging to determine the precise cumulative amount of time spent exercising during an intervention. In the trials that were analysed, a single exercise session might last anywhere between 10 minutes to an hour, although exercise programmes typically last 6 to 12 weeks without follow-up after 3, 6, and 12 months. As little as 10 minutes of exercise three times a week has been shown to have positive effects [165].

Type:

Active exercise as the form of strengthening and/or endurance exercises is advised in addition to stretching, coordination, centralization techniques, nerve mobilisations, traction, manual treatment, patient education, and counseling. Exercises for building endurance are especially helpful since the deep neck flexors at the level of the cervical spine, which are important for stabilising the neck during posture maintenance, are frequently impacted by chronic neck pain [166]. It was seldom recognised that resistance and endurance exercises were a part of the same workout programme; instead, the efficiency of the various activities was directly compared. Numerous research evaluated here included aerobic exercise, which led to an improvement in patient satisfaction, perceptions of health-related quality of life, and overall perceived benefits. Despite not being frequently researched, Jull et al.'s study on the potential advantages of proprioceptive exercises with joint position training discovered that joint position error had been statistically considerably reduced. When compared to a craniocervical flexion training programme, there were also positive outcomes for decreased disability and pain scores for the same training group. Consequently, including 1 of them in an exercise programme might result in positive results [167].

A family of gentle osteopathic manipulation methods known as muscle energy techniques (MET) uses guided and regulated patient-initiated isometric and isotonic contractions to enhance musculoskeletal function and lessen discomfort. Post-isometric relaxation (PIR) is a technique that involves isometrically contracting hyperactive muscles for a short while, followed by a brief latent period of relaxation to allow for gradual muscular lengthening [168]. In accordance with Chaitow, MET consists of an engaged isometric contraction technique combined with moist heat therapy that loosens the muscle and restores normal blood as well as lymphatic circulation by modifying the interstitial pressure as well as trans-capillary circulation that aids in washing away nociceptive stimulants that cause pain to subside. Due to changes in the muscle's viscoelastic properties, MET with PIR aids in reducing muscular tension and increasing muscle flexibility. In the discipline of physiotherapy, procedures like static stretching and muscular energy techniques are frequently employed. MET is a sophisticated stretching method. Studies comparing these two procedures with a symptomatic population have shown contradictory findings, however, studies comparing these two techniques for symptomatic persons have shown improvement in both symptomatic and asymptomatic individuals [169].

Lower Extremity Disorders (including Knee Joint)

One of the most prevalent diseases in the community is pain around the knee joints. All ages are susceptible to chronic knee discomfort, but the elderly are more susceptible. According to studies, over 25 percent of people over 55 have chronic pain in one or both knees, and this is typically accompanied with impairment, especially when it comes to weight-bearing functional chores.The great majority of this knee pain in people over the age of 38 is attributed to osteoarthritis, which radiological symptoms are quite common in the community and sharply increase with advancing age. Although these radiographic alterations are frequently asymptomatic, symptomatic knee osteoarthritis continues to be the most common disease-related cause of reliance in lower limb duties, particularly in the elderly, with a projected incidence of 240 in 100 000 person years [170].

Disorder	Description
Anterior Cruciate Ligament (ACL) Tear	ACL tears often result from sudden stops, changes in direction, or direct impact during activities common in sports professionals, especially athletes involved in sports such as soccer, basketball, or football.
Plantar Fasciitis	Prolonged standing or walking on hard surfaces during occupations like retail, healthcare, or factory work can contribute to plantar fasciitis.
Achilles Tendonitis/Tendinopathy	Occupations requiring repetitive actions like running, jumping, or physically demanding tasks, such as construction work or military service, may lead to Achilles tendonitis.
Patellofemoral Pain Syndrome (PFPS)	PFPS is common in individuals with occupations involving frequent kneeling, squatting, or climbing stairs, including occupations in construction, plumbing, or flooring.
Ankle Sprains	Occupations involving uneven surfaces or requiring rapid changes in direction, such as landscaping, firefighting, or athletics, increase the risk of ankle sprains.
Sciatica and Lumbar Disc Herniation	Jobs involving prolonged sitting, heavy lifting, or improper body mechanics, such as truck driving, construction, or jobs with frequent lifting, may contribute to sciatica and lumbar disc herniation.
Knee Pain and Osteoarthritis (OA))	Repetitive stress on the knee joint from activities like heavy lifting, prolonged kneeling, or repetitive bending seen in occupations like construction, agriculture, or manual labor can lead to knee pain and osteoarthritis over time.

Figure 15: Summary of Occupational Lower Extremity Disorders

Anterior Cruciate Ligament (ACL) Tear

Following an ACL tear, physiotherapy plays a vital role in pre-operative and post-operative care. Pre-operatively, it aims to reduce swelling, restore range of motion, and strengthen supporting muscles. Post-operatively, rehabilitation focuses on regaining knee stability through progressive exercises, proprioception training, and neuromuscular control. Functional training is emphasized for a safe return to sports or daily activities [165].

Plantar Fasciitis

Plantar fasciitis involves pain and inflammation of the heel and arch of the foot. Physiotherapy employs stretching and strengthening exercises for the calf muscles and plantar fascia. Manual therapy techniques enhance tissue mobility, and modalities like ultrasound or shockwave therapy may be used for pain relief. Customized orthotics or footwear recommendations may also be provided for long-term management [166].

Achilles Tendonitis/Tendinopathy

Achilles tendon disorders require a specialized physiotherapy approach. Eccentric strengthening exercises are fundamental in the rehabilitation process. Modalities such as ultrasound and shockwave therapy promote tissue healing. Gait analysis and correction may be employed to reduce stress on the Achilles tendon. A comprehensive program aims to restore strength, flexibility, and function [167].

Patellofemoral Pain Syndrome (PFPS)

PFPS presents as knee pain, particularly around the patella (kneecap). Physiotherapy focuses on strengthening the quadriceps, hip abductors, and gluteal muscles to improve patellar tracking. Manual therapy techniques and taping may be used to alleviate pain and improve joint mechanics. Gait retraining and movement pattern correction are essential components of treatment, aiming to restore pain-free movement [168].

Ankle Sprains

Ankle sprains are common injuries that benefit from physiotherapeutic intervention. Initially, RICE (Rest, Ice, Compression, Elevation) is applied, followed by a range of motion and proprioceptive exercises. Strengthening exercises for the ankle stabilizing muscles are gradually introduced. Balance training and agility drills help restore functional stability, reducing the risk of re-injury [169].

Sciatica and Lumbar Disc Herniation

Sciatica, often associated with lumbar disc herniation, involves radiating pain down the leg due to nerve compression. Physiotherapy includes lumbar spine mobilization, core stabilization, and sciatic nerve gliding exercises. Modalities like heat, TENS, or ultrasound may be used for pain relief. Education on posture, body mechanics, and ergonomics is crucial for long-term management. A tailored program aims to alleviate pain and improve function [170].

Knee Pain and Osteoarthritis (OA)

Knee Osteoarthritis is a degenerative joint disease, characterized by loss of articular cartilage followed by periarticular bone remodeling. The American College of Rheumatology describes Osteoarthritis as a heterogeneous group of conditions that leads to joint symptoms and signs that are associated with defective integrity of articular cartilage, in addition to related changes in the underlying bone at the joint margins. Osteoarthritis is found to be the major etiology of knee pain, especially in people over 55 [170-173]. In fact, using the American College of Rheumatology's widest classification criteria, everyone over 40 with knee discomfort and morning stiffness lasting fewer than 30 minutes would be diagnosed with osteoarthritis of the knee. Focal cartilage loss coupled with a bone "reaction," such as osteophytosis, sclerosis, cyst development, or attrition, are the histological characteristics of osteoarthritis. The radiographic knee osteoarthritis grading system created by Lawrence during the 1950s takes these characteristics into account. Although the scale method has been improved, and the radiography procedure has been standardised, the fundamentals of this system of ratings are still used today [171]. This method's application to different radiological views regarding the knee, such as skyline and lateral views, as well as the patellofemoral compartment, is one of its possible benefits. While X-rays predominantly detect bone, magnetic resonance imaging (MRI) studies show that the soft tissue structures in knee osteoarthritis bear the burden of the degenerative processes. Therefore, MRI has several benefits as a research technique for examining the prevalence and progression of knee osteoarthritis [172]. Figure 16 shows the stages of OA.

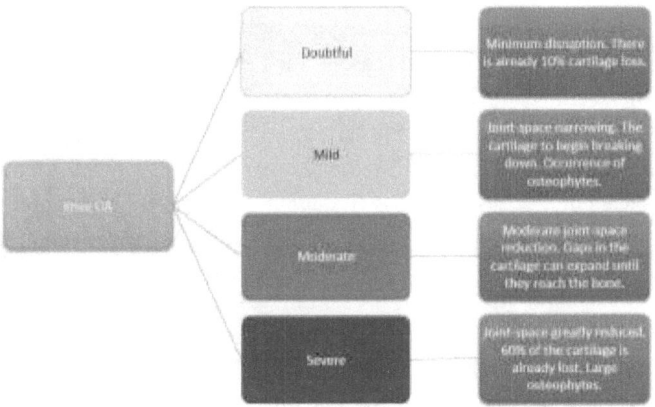

Figure 16: The stages of OA according to its severity

Chondromalacia

Chronic anterior knee discomfort along with characteristic alterations in the patellar articular cartilage define the clinical diagnosis known as chondromalacia patellae. Nevertheless, chondromalacia seems to be widespread, especially in children and teenagers as well as people who engage in specific strenuous sports. People who have chondromalacia patellae may be a subgroup of the wider population of people who experience "anterior knee pain," a chronic pain illness that is generally idiopathic. However, specific investigation of a retro patellar cartilage problem is essential for the accurate diagnosis of chondromalacia patellae. This is often done by arthroscopy. Chondromalacia patellae has an unknown aetiology. It is believed that overuse and mechanical variables like patella alta and irregular patellar tracking play a significant role in fostering the development of a knee joint [173].

Internal alterations

The knee contains a wide range of different soft tissue components that might be implicated as sporadic causes of persistent knee pain. Certain types of knee pain are frequently attributed to mechanical reasons such as ligamentous "strains," meniscal tears, bursitis, popliteal "cysts," iliotibial band syndrome, and synovial plicae. Plicae are incompletely resorbing mesenchymal remains that leave synovial tissue pleats at various locations throughout the knee. They're quite common and mostly unimportant, although they can swell and cause discomfort, crepitus, cracking, and effusion [174].

Other sources of knee discomfort

There are several illnesses that, while being uncommon causes of knee discomfort in the general population, ought to be investigated since they call for a proper diagnosis and course of action. The most frequent of them are synovitis brought on by a crystal-mediated illness like gout or a systemic inflammatory joint disorder like rheumatoid arthritis. Spontaneous osteonecrosis in the knee or pigmented villonodular synovitis are two additional serious conditions. The disease in the hip joint or the lumbar spine, for example, may be the cause of pain felt in the knee [175].

Chronic regional pain syndrome is knee osteoarthritis

The classic disease process paradigm has consistently been challenged by the poor degree of agreement between the pathological alterations of knee osteoarthritis and the effect of the illness, in terms of both pain and disability. Numerous investigations have shown that individual diversity in clinical outcomes is not greatly influenced by the degree of osteoarthritis pathology. The impact of scientific knee osteoarthritis may also be predicted by a number of behavioural and psychological aspects more accurately than by the degree of damage seen in the joint, according to a substantial body of research [176].

Knee osteoarthritis incidence and prevalence

The frequency of knee discomfort in the general population rises with ageing. regarding 30% of people over the age of 40 who participated in surveys regarding population samples report having chronic pain in one or both knees. According to population surveys, one-third of adults over 63 show radiographic signs of osteoarthritis in their knee joints, which suggests that a large portion of the community's chronic knee discomfort is caused by osteoarthritis [177]. Since many cases of radiographic knee osteoarthritis are asymptomatic as well as conversely, a portion of symptomatic people possess normal radiographic appearances, prevalence estimates for symptomatic osteoarthritis of the knee (i.e. persistent pain in the knee accompanied with radiographic signs of osteoarthritis) are lower in practice. Therefore, according to epidemiological studies, the incidence of symptomatic knee osteoarthritis varies from 1.6% to 9.5% depending on the age distribution of the sample, with larger rates seen in older individuals. The bulk of these investigations, it should be highlighted, only got tibiofemoral views and likely missed occasions with lone patellofemoral osteoarthritis, which is a significant contributor to pain and impairment. Women had greater rates than males, especially beyond the age of 50, and the prevalence rose with age [177,178]. The pathophysiology of OA has been illustrated in Figure 17.

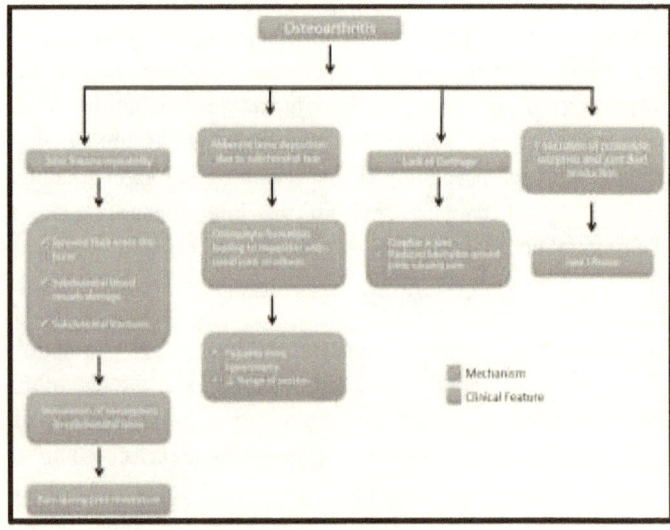

Figure 17: Pathophysiology of OA

Physiotherapy management

Physiotherapy plays a crucial role in the management of osteoarthritis (OA). A physiotherapist can design a tailored exercise and treatment plan to help alleviate pain, improve joint function, and enhance the overall quality of life for individuals with OA [178].

Exercise

Exercise treatment is recognised as the foundation of conservative care and is advised by clinical guidelines due to the substantial body of data indicating the positive therapeutic benefits of exercise in persons with knee OA of varied severity. Importantly, unlike medications and surgery, exercise comes with minimal contraindications and negative side effects while still having similar effect sizes to basic analgesic and non-steroidal anti-inflammatory treatments [179]. Due to decreased physical activity and pain management, people who have knee OA frequently have decreased muscular strength. The quadriceps have the greatest capacity to produce and absorb stresses at the knee since they are the biggest set of muscles to traverse the knee joint. Numerous clinical investigations have demonstrated that training consistently increases knee extension strength and decreases pain and physical impairment in individuals with knee OA. However, it hasn't been found that one kind of strength training is better than another [180]. Although a mix of strengthening, aerobic, and functional exercise is advised, there is currently no data to support the benefit of one particular style of exercise over another. Additionally, exercise can be given through private sessions, supervised group groups, or at home [178-181]. It seems that all three methods of exercise administration are successful in lowering symptoms; however, interaction with a therapist could lead to better results. The frequency and length of an exercise programme are other factors. Exercise programmes in people with knee OA have improved symptoms after 8–12 weeks, according to the majority of exercise guidelines, and physiological effects can be achieved with as little as 2-3 exercise sessions per week. The ideal exercise dose must be individualised for every patient and is still to be found [181].

In the initial few months after starting an exercise programme, adherence to exercising is frequently strong, but it quickly falls with time. In individuals who have knee OA, improvement in outcomes from exercise treatment depends critically on patient adherence. Patients who get attention from medical professionals, trust in the efficacy of the intervention and comprehend the aetiology of knee OA adhere better. Self-efficacy, or confidence in one's own capacity to carry out activities, is likewise linked to higher levels of adherence and superior results [182].

Taping

According to certain professional standards, physiotherapy treatment for knee OA includes taping the knee, especially the patella. Applying sticky stiff strapping tape to a patella and/or other nearby soft tissue structures is known as knee taping. The ultimate goal of taping is to relieve uncomfortable soft tissues surrounding the knee joint and reposition the patella to alleviate stress on the patellofemoral joint (PFJ) [180,181]. Numerous randomised controlled trials in individuals with knee OA, both with and without OA of the PFJ, have shown immediate and short-term decreases in pain. Although the exact process by which tape lowers pain is unknown, it may involve adjustments to the patellar alignment26 as well as improved muscle function and activation [183].

Bracing

For knee OA, there are several commercial braces that vary in terms of cost, build, and design. A single-piece sleeve constructed from neoprene is the most basic design, and there is proof that it helps lessen discomfort. Unicompartmental OA can be treated with an "unloader knee brace." It is a molded plastic and foam brace with metal side columns that is semi-rigid and frequently produced to order. By shifting stress away from the troublesome side, the brace's design seeks to alter how force circulates at the knee, and biomechanical studies back up this load-reducing effect. Numerous clinical studies on these braces reveal symptomatic advantages for people with unicompartmental OA, however, the impact may vary depending on the individual patient and brace. In obese patients, braces have been shown to have been less effective, and 'off the shelf' designs were found to be inferior to custom-made ones [184].

Adherence is probably one of the main obstacles preventing a brace treatment for knee OA from providing its full advantages. Bulkiness, style, simplicity of application, fit, and comfort are just a few examples of factors that might contribute to poor adherence. A brace shouldn't be used for a stand-alone treatment for osteoarthritis because there isn't enough data on its efficacy, and the choice to use one should be dependent on how each patient responds [185].

Shoes and Insoles

Shoes and insoles have a lot of potential as quick, low-cost therapy options for knee OA. For lateral compartment disease and medial compartment OA, lateral wedge insoles are recommended. According to biomechanical research, in medial knee OA, lateral wedges lessen the adduction moment when walking by 4-12% when compared to wearing bare feet or only shoes. As a result, the medial compartment burden is decreased. Knee load is influenced by footwear, and the current study indicates that specific shoe qualities may have an effect. It suggests that stable, more supporting shoes increase knee stress, whereas flexible footwear and footwear with a heel height of less than 38 mm reduce knee load [186].

Manual treatment

Joint manipulation and mobilisation are among the various procedures used in manual therapy, and they are by far the most popular. While manipulation is described as powerful small-amplitude, high-velocity motions of a joint often administered at the end of the range, mobilisation is a manual approach that uses repetitive passive movements of low velocity and varied amplitudes. According to studies, manual therapy is often utilised in clinical practise for OA, with 96% of Irish therapists and 64% of all UK therapists using it to treat those suffering from knee and hip OA, respectively [185-187].

Overall, the main physiotherapy that can be applied in osteoarthritis has been summarized in Figure 18.

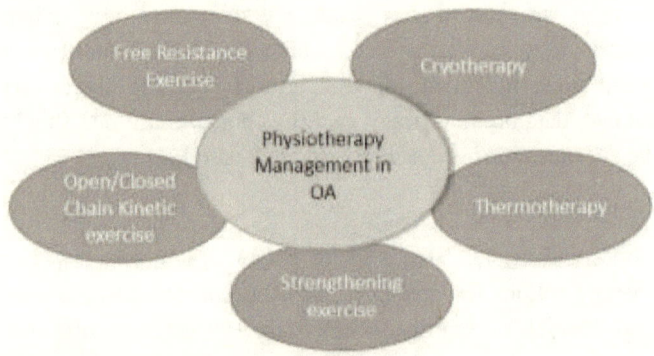

Figure 18: Physiotherapy Management in osteoarthritis

Workplace prevention tips for each condition

Cervical Syndrome: Ergonomic workstations can help reduce the risk of cervical syndrome in the workplace [5]. Use ergonomic chairs, raise computer screens to a comfortable viewing height, and get up and move around every so often. Raise awareness of the problem and encourage staff to do neck exercises to alleviate pressure.

Thoracic Outlet Syndrome: Maintain ergonomic workstations, promote proper posture, and extend shoulders to prevent Thoracic Outlet Syndrome at work [23]. To reduce thoracic outlet nerve and blood vessel compression, encourage employees to take breaks, vary duties, and avoid prolonged overhead activity.

Shoulder Tendinitis and Capsulitis: Avoid shoulder tendonitis and capsulitis at work by using ergonomic workstations, shoulder-friendly workouts, and proper lifting techniques. Encourage stretching breaks and posture education to reduce strain. These techniques prevent shoulder tendon and joint capsule irritation and injury.

Carpal Tunnel Syndrome: Keep wrists neutral, use ergonomic tools, and stretch regularly to avoid Carpal Tunnel Syndrome at work. Place keyboards and mice properly and encourage hand exercises [12]. These treatments lower median nerve pressure, reducing Carpal Tunnel Syndrome risk.

Medial epicondylitis: Use ergonomic tools, gripping techniques, and forearm exercises to prevent medial epicondylitis at work. Use diversified chores and pauses to reduce repetitive motions. By strengthening forearm muscles, inner elbow tendon tension can be avoided.

Posterior Interosseous Nerve Syndrome: Avoid repetitive twisting, use ergonomic tools, and stretch your hands and wrists to prevent Posterior Interosseous Nerve Syndrome at work [186]. Proper hand alignment and short rests lessen posterior interosseous nerve compression, preventing nerve disorders.

Forearm Myalgia: Forearm myalgia can be prevented at work by using ergonomic workstations, taking microbreaks for stretches, and varying tasks. Promote good typing and gripping methods and strengthen forearm muscles with tailored exercises. These techniques reduce muscular fatigue and strain, lowering forearm myalgia risk.

De Quervains: Use ergonomic gear, thumb-friendly hand positions, and thumb stretches to prevent De Quervains at work [1]. To lessen thumb motions, take breaks and switch tasks. These strategies reduce occupational tenosynovitis by protecting thumb tendons.

Extensor Tenosynovitis: Workplace extensor tenosynovitis can be prevented by switching duties, good hand placement, and wrist stretches. Reduce repetitive hand and wrist motions with ergonomic tools and breaks. Strengthen forearm muscles to support extensor tendons and reduce inflammation.

Osteoarthritis: Workplace osteoarthritis can be prevented by using joint-friendly gear, good posture, and low-impact activities [187]. To prevent workplace-related osteoarthritis, encourage employees to take breaks, stretch, and maintain a healthy weight.

References

1. Korhonen T, Ketola R, Toivonen R, Luukkonen R, Häkkänen M, Viikari-Juntura E: Work related and individual predictors for incident neck pain among office employees working with video display units. Occup Environ Med. 2003, 60:475-82. 10.1136/oem.60.7.475.

2. De Loose V, Burnotte F, Cagnie B, Stevens V, Van Tiggelen D: Prevalence and risk factors of neck pain in military office workers. Mil Med. 2008, 173:474-9. 10.7205/milmed.173.5.474.

3. Shannon HS, Woodward CA, Cunningham CE, McIntosh J, Lendrum B, Brown J, Rosenbloom D: Changes in general health and musculoskeletal outcomes in the workforce of a hospital undergoing rapid change: a longitudinal study. J

Occup Health Psychol. 2001, 6:3-14. 10.1037//1076-8998.6.1.3.

4. Hoe VC, Urquhart DM, Kelsall HL, Zamri EN, Sim MR: Ergonomic interventions for preventing work-related musculoskeletal disorders of the upper limb and neck among office workers. Cochrane Database Syst Rev. 2018, 10:CD008570. 10.1002/14651858.CD008570.pub3.

5. Westgaard RH, Winkel J: Ergonomic intervention research for improved musculoskeletal health: a critical review. Centre for Reviews and Dissemination. 1997,

6. O'Riordan C, Clifford A, Van De Ven P, Nelson J: Chronic neck pain and exercise interventions: frequency, intensity, time, and type principle. Arch Phys Med Rehabil. 2014, 95:770-83. 10.1016/j.apmr.2013.11.015.

7. Letafatkar A, Rabiei P, Alamooti G, Bertozzi L, Farivar N, Afshari M: Effect of therapeutic exercise routine on pain, disability, posture, and health status in dentists with chronic neck pain: a randomized controlled trial. Int Arch Occup Environ Health. 2020, 93:281-90. 10.1007/s00420-019-01480-x.

8. Shariat A, Cleland JA, Danaee M, Kargarfard M, Sangelaji B, Tamrin SB: Effects of stretching exercise training and ergonomic modifications on musculoskeletal discomforts of office workers: a randomized controlled trial. Braz J Phys Ther. 2018, 22:144-53. 10.1016/j.bjpt.2017.09.003.

9. Fabrizio P: Ergonomic intervention in the treatment of a patient with upper extremity and neck pain . Phys Ther. 2009, 89:351-60. 10.2522/ptj.20080209 15. Chen X, Coombes BK, Sjøgaard G, Jun D, O'Leary S, Johnston V: Workplace-based interventions for neck pain in office workers: systematic

review and meta-analysis. Phys Ther. 2018, 98:40-62. 10.1093/ptj/pzx101.

10. Aaras, A., Ro, O., 1997. Workload when using a mouse as an input (device. Int. J. Hum.–Comput. Interact. 9, 105–118.

11. Aaras, A., Ro, O., Thorensen, M., 1999. Can a more neutral position (of the forearm when operating a computer mouse reduce the pain level for visual display unit operators? A prospective epidemiological intervention study. Int. J. Hum.–Comput. Interact. 11, 79–94.

12. Armstrong, T., Castelli, W., Evans, G., Dias-Perez, R., 1984. Some histological changes in carpal tunnel contents and their biomechanical implications. J. Occup. Med. 26, 197–201.

13. Armstrong, T.J., Buckle, P., Fine, L.J., Hagberg, M., Jonsson, B., Kilbom, A., Kuorinka, I., Silverstein, B.A., Sjogaard, G., Viikari- (Juntura, E., 1993. A conceptual model for work-related neck and upper-limbmusculoskeletal disorders. Scand. J. Work Environ. Health 19, 73–84.

14. Ashton-Miller, J.A., 1999. Response of muscle and tendon to injury and overuse. Work-related Musculoskeletal Disorders: Report, Workshop Summary, and Workshop Papers, National Research Council. National Academy Press, Washington, DC, pp. 73–97.

15. Besson, J., 1999. The neurobiology of pain. Lancet 353, 1610–1615.

16. Blair, S., 1996. Pathophysiology of cumulative trauma disorders: some possible humoral and nervous system mechanisms. In: Moon, S.D., Sauter, S.L. (Eds.), Beyond Biomechanics: Psychosocial Aspects of Musculoskeletal Disorders in Office Work. Taylor and Francis, London, pp. 91–97.

17. Franzblau A, Werner RA. What is carpal tunnel syndrome? JAMA. 1999; 282:186–187.

18. Gerr F, Letz R. The sensitivity and specificity of tests for carpal tunnel syndrome vary with the comparison groups. J Hand Surg. 1998; 23-B:151–155.

19. Szabo RM, Slater RR, Farver TB, Stanton DB, Sharman WK. The value of diagnostic testing in carpal tunnel syndrome. J Hand Surg. 1999; 24-A:704–714.

20. Ferry S, Pritchard T, Keenan J, et al. Estimating the prevalence of delayed median nerve conduction in the general population. Br J Rheumatol. 1998; 37:630–635.

21. The American Academy of Electrodiagnostic Medicine; The American Academy of Neurology; The American Academy of Physical Medicine and Rehabilitation. Practice parameters for electrodiagnosis in carpal tunnel syndrome: summary statement. Muscle Nerve. 1993; 16:1390–1391.

22. Nordstrom DL, Vierkant RA, DeStefano F, Layde PM. Risk factors for carpal tunnel syndrome in a general population. Occup Environ Med. 1997; 54:734–740.

23. Solomon DH, Katz JN, Bohn R, et al. Non-occupational risk factors for carpal tunnel syndrome. J Gen Intern Med. 1999; 14:310–314.

24. Hagberg M, Morgenstern H, Kelsh M. Impact of occupations and job tasks on the prevalence of carpal tunnel syndrome. Scand J Work Environ Health. 1992; 18:337–345.

25. National Institute for Occupational Health and Safety. A Critical Review of Epidemiologic Evidence for Work-Related Musculoskeletal Disorders of the Neck, Upper Extremity, and Low Back. US Department of Health and Human Sciences/NIOSH; Cincinnati, OH: 1997. Musculoskeletal Disorders and Workplace Factors. Publication no. 97-141.

26. Abbas MAF, Afifi AA, Zhang ZW, Kraus JF. Meta-analysis of published studies of work-related carpal tunnel syndrome. Int J Occup Environ Health. 1998; 4:160–167. [PubMed: 10026477] 16. Palmer KT, Harris EC, Coggon D. Carpal tunnel syndrome and its relation to occupation: a systematic literature review. Occup Med. 2007; 57:57–66.

27. Thomsen JF, Gerr F, Atroshi I. Carpal tunnel syndrome and the use of computer mouse and keyboard: a systematic review. BMC Musculoskeletal Disorders. 2008; 9:134.

28. Mediouni Z, de Roquemaurel A, Dumontier C, et al. Is carpal tunnel syndrome related to computer exposure at work? A review and meta-analysis. J Occup Environ Med. 2014; 56:204–208.

29. Page MJ, Massy-Westropp N, O'Connor D, Pitt V. Splinting for carpal tunnel syndrome. Cochrane Database Syst Rev. Jul 11.2012 7:CD010003. doi: 10.1002/14651858.CD010003.

30. Piazzini DB, Aprile I, Ferrara PE, et al. A systematic review of conservative treatment of carpal tunnel syndrome. Clin Rehabil. 2007; 21(4):299–314.

31. Graham B. Nonsurgical treatment of carpal tunnel syndrome. J Hand Surg Am. 2009; 34(3):531–4.

32. O'Connor D, Marshall SC, Massy-Westropp N, Pitt V. Non-surgical treatment (other than steroid injection) for carpal tunnel syndrome. Cochrane Database Syst Rev. Jan 20.2003 :CD003219.

33. Marshall S, Tardif G, Ashworth N. Local corticosteroid injection for carpal tunnel syndrome. Cochrane Database Syst Rev. Apr 18.2007 :CD001554.

34. Ebenbichler GR, Resch KL, Nicolakis P, et al. Ultrasound treatment for treating the carpal tunnel syndrome: randomised 'sham' controlled trial. BMJ. 1998; 316:731–5.

35. Baker NA, Livengood HM. Symptom severity and conservative treatment for carpal tunnel syndrome in association with eventual carpal tunnel release. J Hand Surg [Am]. 2014; 39:1792–98.

36. Amadio P. The Mayo Clinic and carpal tunnel syndrome. Mayo Clin Proc. 1992; 67:42–8.

37. Iliev A, Jelev L, Landzhov B, Malinova L, Hinova-Palova D, Paloff A, Ovtscharoff W: A doubled palmaris longus muscle: case report. Acta Morphol Anthropol. 2012, 19:78-80.

38. Kotov G, Iliev A, Georgiev GP, Karabinov V, Landzhov B: Clinical significance of anatomical variations in the carpal tunnel: review. Acta Morphol Anthropol. 2017, 24:109-113.

39. Target radio frequency therapy - history, development and application. (Content in Bulgarian). (2017). Accessed: March 3 ,2020:

40. Graham B, Peljovich A, Afra R, et al.: The American Academy of Orthopaedic Surgeons Evidence-Based Clinical Practice Guideline on: Management of Carpal Tunnel Syndrome. J Bone Joint Surg Am. 2016, 98:1750-1754. 10.2106/JBJS.16.00719.

41. Martins RS, Siqueira MG: Conservative therapeutic management of carpal tunnel syndrome . Arq Neuropsiquiatr. 2017, 75:819-824.

42. Kostadinov D, Gacheva Y, Tsvetkova D: Physical therapy manual . Kostadinov D (ed): Medicina i Fizkultura, Sofia, Bulgaria; 1989.

43. Kostadinov D: Physiotherapy. Kostadinov D (ed): Medicina i Fizkultura, Sofia, Bulgaria; 1991.

44. Rempel 1999 {published data only} Rempel D, Tittiranonda P, Burastero S, Hudes M, So Y. Effect of keyboard keyswitch design on hand pain. Journal of Occupational and Environmental Medicine 1999;41(2): 111–9.

45. Andersson GBJ (1999) Epidemiological features of chronic low back pain. Lancet 354, 581–585. Arad D and Ryan M (1986) The incidence and prevalence in nurses of low back pain: a definitive survey exposes the hazards. Australian Nurse Journal 16, 44–48.

46. Cheung K (2010) The incidence of low back problems among nursing students in Hong Kong. Journal of Clinical Nursing 19, 2355–2362.

47. Cooper C, Coggon D, Smedley J, Trevelyan F, Inskip H and Buckle P (2003) Impact of ergonomic intervention on back pain among nurses. Scandinav Journal of Work Environment and Health 29, 117–123.

48. Cunningham C, Flynn T and Blake C (2006) Low back pain and occupation among Irish health service workers. Occupational Medicine (London) 56, 447–454.

49. Deyo RA and Weinstein JN (2001) Low back pain. The New England Journal of Medicine 344, 363–370.

50. Tittiranonda 1999 {published data only} Tittiranonda P, Rempel D, Armstrong T, Burastero S. Effect of four computer keyboards in computer users with upper extremity musculoskeletal disorders. American Journal of Industrial Medicine 1999;35(6):647–61.

51. Andersen 2003 {published data only} Andersen JH, Thomsen JF, Overgaard E, Lassen CF, Brandt LPA, Vilstrup I, et al. Computer use and carpal tunnel syndrome: a 1-year

follow-up study. JAMA: Journal of the American Medical Association 2003;289(22):2963–9.

52. Woo SL, Lee TQ, Abramowitch SD, et al. Structure and function of ligaments and tendons. In: Mow VC, Huiskes R, editors. Basic Orthopaedic Biomechanics and Mechanobiology. Philadelphia: Lippincott, Williams and Wilkins; 2005. p. 301–42.

53. Barr AE, Barbe MF, Clark BD. Work-related musculoskeletal disorders of the hand and wrist: epidemiology, pathophysiology, and sensorimotor changes. J Orthop Sports Phys Ther 2004;34(10):610–27.

54. Gruchow HW, Pelletier D. An epidemiologic study of tennis elbow. Incidence, recurrence, and effectiveness of prevention strategies. Am J Sports Med 1979; 7(4):234–8.

55. James SL, Bates BT, Osternig LR. Injuries to runners. Am J Sports Med 1978;6(2): 40–50.

56. Bare AA, Haddad SL. Tenosynovitis of the posterior tibial tendon. Foot Ankle Clin 2001;6(1):37–66.

57. Rogier C, Hayer S, van der Helm-van Mil A. Not only synovitis but also tenosynovitis needs to be considered: why it is time to update textbook images of rheumatoid arthritis. Ann Rheum Dis. 2020 Apr;79(4):546-547.

58. Hayer S, Redlich K, Korb A, Hermann S, Smolen J, Schett G. Tenosynovitis and osteoclast formation as the initial preclinical changes in a murine model of inflammatory arthritis. Arthritis Rheum. 2007 Jan;56(1):79-88.

59. McQueen F, Lassere M, Østergaard M. Magnetic resonance imaging in psoriatic arthritis: a review of the literature. Arthritis Res Ther. 2006;8(2):207.

60. Chen S, Chen M, Wu X, Lin S, Tao C, Cao H, Shao Z, Xiao G. Global, regional and national burden of low back pain 1990-2019: A systematic analysis of the Global Burden of Disease study 2019. J Orthop Translat. 2021 Sep 10;32:49-58. doi: 10.1016/j.jot.2021.07.005. PMID: 34934626; PMCID: PMC8639804.

61. Cagliero E, Apruzzese W, Perlmutter GS, Nathan DM. Musculoskeletal disorders of the hand and shoulder in patients with diabetes mellitus. Am J Med. 2002 Apr 15;112(6):487-90.

62. Strom L. Trigger finger in diabetes. J Med Soc N J. 1977 Nov;74(11):951-4.

63. Giladi AM, Malay S, Chung KC. A systematic review of the management of acute pyogenic flexor tenosynovitis. J Hand Surg Eur Vol. 2015 Sep;40(7):720-8.

64. Gray RG, Gottlieb NL. Hand flexor tenosynovitis in rheumatoid arthritis. Prevalence, distribution, and associated rheumatic features. Arthritis Rheum. 1977 May;20(4):1003-8.

65. Adams JE, Habbu R. Tendinopathies of the Hand and Wrist. J Am Acad Orthop Surg. 2015 Dec;23(12):741-50.

66. Adams JE, Habbu R. Tendinopathies of the Hand and Wrist. J Am Acad Orthop Surg 2015; 23(12): 741-750.

67. Cavaleri R, Schabrun SM, Te M, Chipchase LS. Hand therapy versus corticosteroid injections in the treatment of de Quervain's disease: A systematic review and meta-analysis. J Hand Ther 2016; 29(1): 3-11.

68. Huisstede BM, Gladdines S, Randsdorp MS, Koes BW. Effectiveness of conservative, surgical, and post-surgical interventions for Trigger finger, Dupuytren's disease, and De Quervain's disease. A systematic review. Arch Phys Med Rehabil 2017.

69. Niethard FU, Pfeil J, Biberthaler P. Duale Reihe Orthopädie und Unfallchirurgie. Stuttgart: Thieme; 2014.

70. Peters-Veluthamaningal C, van der Windt DA, Winters JC, Meyboom-de Jong B. Corticosteroid injection for de Quervain's tenosynovitis. Cochrane Database Syst Rev 2009; (3): CD005616.

71. Peters-Veluthamaningal C, van der Windt DA, Winters JC, Meyboom-de Jong B. Corticosteroid injection for trigger finger in adults. Cochrane Database Syst Rev 2009; (1): CD005617.

72. Rowland P, Phelan N, Gardiner S, Linton KN, Galvin R. The Effectiveness of Corticosteroid Injection for De Quervain's Stenosing Tenosynovitis (DQST): A Systematic Review and Meta-Analysis. Open Orthop J 2015; 9: 437-444.

73. GBD 2015 Disease and Injury Incidence and Prevalence Collaborators. Global, regional, and national incidence, prevalence, and years lived with disability for 310 diseases and injuries, 1990-2015: a systematic analysis for the Global Burden of Disease Study 2015. Lancet. 2016 Oct 08;388(10053):1545-1602.

74. Jelsma J, Mielke J, Powell G, De Weerdt W, De Cock P. Disability in an urban black community in Zimbabwe. Disabil Rehabil. 2002 Nov 10;24(16):851-9.

75. Fabunmi AA, Aba SO, Odunaiya NA. Prevalence of low back pain among peasant farmers in a rural community in South West Nigeria. Afr J Med Med Sci. 2005 Sep;34(3):259-62.

76. Bass E. Tendinopathy: why the difference between tendinitis and tendinosis matters. Int J Ther Massage Bodywork 2012; 5: 14-17.

77. Malliaras P, Barton CJ, Reeves ND, Langberg H. Achilles and patellar tendinopathy loading programmes : a systematic review comparing clinical outcomes and identifying potential mechanisms for effectiveness. Sports Med 2013; 43: 267-286.

78. Murtaugh B, Ihm JM. Eccentric training for the treatment of tendinopathies. Curr Sports Med Rep 2013; 12: 175-182.

79. Bogduk N. On the definitions and physiology of back pain, referred pain, and radicular pain. Pain. 2009;147:17–9. A delineation of low back pain diagnosis and definition.

80. Atlas SJ, Deyo RA. Evaluating and managing acute low back pain in the primary care setting. J Gen Intern Med, Springer. 2001;16: 120–31.

81. Petering RC, Webb C. Treatment options for low back pain in athletes. Sports Health, SAGE Publications. 2011;3:550–5.

82. Longo UG, Loppini M, Denaro L, Maffulli N, Denaro V. Rating scales for low back pain. Br Med Bull, Oxford University Press. 2010;94:81–144. 5. Lennard T, Vivian D, Walkowski S, Singla A. Pain procedures in clinical practice. Third Edition. Elsevier/Saunders. 2011.

83. Hoy D, March L, Brooks P, Blyth F, Woolf A, Bain C, et al. The global burden of low back pain: estimates from the Global Burden of Disease 2010 study. Ann Rheum Dis, BMJ Publishing Group Ltd. 2014;73:968–74. An epidemiological study of global low back pain burden.

84. Heuch I, Foss IS. Acute low back usually resolves quickly but persistent low back pain often persists. J Physiother. 2013;59:127.

85. American Academy of Family Physicians. TH, Randolph DC. American family physician. Am. Fam. Physician. Leawood: American Academy of Family Physicians; 1970.

86. French SD, Cameron M, Walker BF, Reggars JW, Esterman AJ. Superficial heat or cold for low back pain. Cochrane database Syst Rev, John Wiley and Sons, Ltd. 2006:CD004750.

87. Frerick H, Keitel W, Kuhn U, Schmidt S, Bredehorst A, Kuhlmann M. Topical treatment of chronic low back pain with a capsicum plaster. Pain. 2003;106:59–64.

88. Witenko C, Moorman-Li R, Motycka C, Duane K, HincapieCastillo J, Leonard P, et al. Considerations for the appropriate use of skeletal muscle relaxants for the management of acute low back pain. P T, MediMedia, USA. 2014;39:427–35.

89. American Academy of Family Physicians. AT, Ogle AA. American family physician. Am. Fam. Physician. Leawood: American Academy of Family Physicians; 1970.

90. Samanta J, Kendall J, Samanta A. 10-minute consultation: chronic low back pain. BMJ, British Medical Journal Publishing Group. 2003;326:535.

91. Pincus T, Vlaeyen JWS, Kendall NAS, Von Korff MR, Kalauokalani DA, Reis S. Cognitive-behavioral therapy and psychosocial factors in low back pain: directions for the future. Spine (Phila Pa 1976). 2002;27:E133–8.

92. Elkayam O, Ben Itzhak S, Avrahami E, Meidan Y, Doron N, Eldar I, et al. Multidisciplinary approach to chronic back pain: prognostic elements of the outcome. Clin Exp Rheumatol. 14:281–8.

93. Deyo RA, Weinstein JN. Low Back Pain. N Engl J Med. 2001;344: 363–70.

94. Deyo RA, Rainville J, Kent DL. What can the history and physical examination tell us about low back pain? JAMA J Am Med Assoc, American Medical Association. 1992;268:760.

95. Chou R. Low back pain. Ann Intern Med, American College of Physicians. 2014;160:ITC6–1. An overview of low back pain.

96. Theis JL, Finkelstein MJ. Long-term effects of safe patient handling program on staff injuries. Rehabil Nurs. 2014 Jan-Feb;39(1):26-35.

97. Anyan W, Faraklas I, Morris S, Cochran A. Overhead lift systems reduce back injuries among burn care providers. J Burn Care Res. 2013 Nov-Dec;34(6):586-90.

98. Schoenfisch AL, Lipscomb HJ, Myers DJ, Fricklas E, James T. A lift assist team in an acute care hospital-prevention of injury or transfer of risk during patient-handling tasks? AAOHN J. 2011 Aug;59(8):329-34.

99. Kindblom-Rising K, Wahlström R, Nilsson-Wikmar L, Buer N. Nursing staff's movement awareness, attitudes and reported behaviour in patient transfer before and after an educational intervention. Appl Ergon. 2011 Mar;42(3):455-63.

100. Garg A, Kapellusch JM. Long-term efficacy of an ergonomics program that includes patient-handling devices on reducing musculoskeletal injuries to nursing personnel. Hum Factors. 2012 Aug;54(4):608-25.

101. Al-Tannir MA, Kobrosly SY, Elbakri NK, Abu-Shaheen AK. Prevalence and predictors of physical exercise among nurses. A cross-sectional study. Saudi Med J. 2017 Feb;38(2):209-212.

102. Nicholls R, Perry L, Duffield C, Gallagher R, Pierce H. Barriers and facilitators to healthy eating for nurses in the workplace: an integrative review. J Adv Nurs. 2017 May;73(5):1051-1065.

103. Blake H, Patterson J. Paediatric nurses' attitudes towards the promotion of healthy eating. 2015 Jan 22-Feb 11Br J Nurs. 24(2):108-12.

104. Kyle RG, Wills J, Mahoney C, Hoyle L, Kelly M, Atherton IM. Obesity prevalence among healthcare professionals in England: a cross-sectional study using the Health Survey for England. BMJ Open. 2017 Dec 04;7(12):e018498.

105. Ficarra MG, Gualano MR, Capizzi S, Siliquini R, Liguori G, Manzoli L, Briziarelli L, Parlato A, Cuccurullo P, Bucci R, Piat SC, Masanotti G, de Waure C, Ricciardi W, La Torre G. Tobacco use prevalence, knowledge and attitudes among Italian hospital healthcare professionals. Eur J Public Health. 2011 Feb;21(1):29-34.

106. La Torre G, Tiberio G, Sindoni A, Dorelli B, Cammalleri V. Smoking cessation interventions on health-care workers: a systematic review and meta-analysis. PeerJ. 2020;8:e9396.

107. American Psychiatric Association, Diagnostic and Statistical Manual of Mental Disorders, ed 4. Washington, DC, American Psychiatric Association, 1994, pp 445-470.

108. Ayoub MA, Wittels NE: Cumulative trauma disorders. International Review of Ergoders, ed 4. Washington, DC, American Psychiatric Association, 1994, pp 445-470 nomics 2217-272,1989.

109. Bernard B (ed): Musculoskeletal disorders and workplace factors. Cincinnati, OH, National Institute for Occupational Health and Safety, US Department of Health and Human Services, 1997.

110. Bilgi C, Pelmear PL Hand-arm vibration syndrome: A guide to medical impairment assessment. J Occup Med 35:936-942,1993.

111. Biundo JJ, Mipro RC, Fahey P: Sports-related and other soft-tissue injuries, tendonitis, bursitis, and occupation-related syndromes. Curr Opin Rheumalol9:151-154, 1997.

112. Bovenzi M: Exposure-response relationship in the hand-arm vibration syndrome: An overview of current epidemiology research. Int Arch Occup Environ Health 71:509-519, 1998.

113. Brammer AJ, Taylor W, Lundborg G: Sensorineural stages of the hand-arm vibration syndrome. Scand J Work Environ Health 13:279-283, 1987.

114. Bureau of Labor Statistics: News, United States Department of Labor. Washington, DC, Bureau of Labor Statistics. USDL 99-102, April, 1999.

115. Campbell SM: Regional myofascial pain syndromes. Rheum Dis Clin North Am 15:31- 44,1989.

116. Cohen AL, Gjessing CC, Fine LJ, et al: Elements of Ergonomics Programs. DHHS Publication No. 97-117 Washington, DC, US Department of Health and Human Services, 1997.

117. DeKrom MCTFM, Knipschild PG, Kester ADM: Efficacy of provocative tests for diagnosis of carpal tunnel syndrome. Lancet 335:393-395, 1990.

118. dewinter AF, Jans MP, Scholten RJPM, et al: Diagnostic classification of shoulder disorders: Interobserver agreement and determinants of disagreement. Ann Rheum Dis 58:272-277, 1999.

119. Gemme G, Pyykko I, Taylor W, et al: The Stockholm Workshop scale for the classification of cold-induced Raynauds phenomenon in the hand-arm vibration syndrome (revision of the Taylor-Pelmear scale). Scand J Work Environ Health 13:275-278,1987.

120. Gerr F, Letz R: The sensitivity and specificity of tests for carpal tunnel syndrome vary with the comparison subjects. J Hand Surg [Br123151-155,1998.

121. Hoppenfeld S: Physical Examination of the Spine and Extremities. East Norwalk, CT, Appleton-Century-Crofts, 1976.

122. Katz JN, Lew RA, Bessette L, et al: Prevalence and predictors of long-term work disability due to carpal tunnel syndrome. Am J Ind Med 33:543-550, 1998.

123. LeNoir JL: Subacromial-subdeltoid bursitis of the shoulder. Orthop Rev 730-732, 1986.

124. Luopajarvi T, Kuorinka I, Virolainen M, et al: Prevalence of tenosynovitis and other injuries of the upper extremities in repetitive work. Scand J Work Environ Health 5:48- 55,1979 58:272-277, 1999.

125. Feuerstein M, Nicholas RA: Development of a short form of the workstyle measure . Occup Med (Lond). 2006, 56:94-9. 10.1093/occmed/kqi197

126. Ariëns GA, van Mechelen W, Bongers PM, Bouter LM, van der Wal G: Physical risk factors for neck pain . Scand J Work Environ Health. 2000, 26:7-19. 10.5271/sjweh.504

127. Bernaards CM, Bosmans JE, Hildebrandt VH, van Tulder MW, Heymans MW: The cost-effectiveness of a lifestyle physical activity intervention in addition to a work style intervention on recovery from neck and upper limb symptoms and pain reduction in computer workers. Occup Environ Med. 2011, 68:265-72. 10.1136/oem.2008.045450

128. Barbe MF, Barr AE: Inflammation and the pathophysiology of work-related musculoskeletal disorders . Brain Behav Immun. 2006, 20:423-9. 10.1016/j.bbi.2006.03.001

129. Côté P, van der Velde G, Cassidy JD, et al.: The burden and determinants of neck pain in workers: results of the Bone and Joint Decade 2000-2010 Task Force on Neck Pain and Its Associated Disorders. Spine (Phila Pa 1976). 2008, 33:S60-74. 10.1097/BRS.0b013e3181643ee4

130. Korhonen T, Ketola R, Toivonen R, Luukkonen R, Häkkänen M, Viikari-Juntura E: Work related and individual predictors for incident neck pain among office employees working with video display units. Occup Environ Med. 2003, 60:475-82. 10.1136/oem.60.7.475

131. De Loose V, Burnotte F, Cagnie B, Stevens V, Van Tiggelen D: Prevalence and risk factors of neck pain in military office workers. Mil Med. 2008, 173:474-9. 10.7205/milmed.173.5.474

132. Shannon HS, Woodward CA, Cunningham CE, McIntosh J, Lendrum B, Brown J, Rosenbloom D: Changes in general health and musculoskeletal outcomes in the workforce of a hospital undergoing rapid change: a longitudinal study. J Occup Health Psychol. 2001, 6:3-14. 10.1037//1076-8998.6.1.3

133. Moore JS: Carpal tunnel syndrome. Occup Med 7:741-763,1992.

134. Moore JS: Function, structure, and responses of components of the muscle-tendon unit.

135. Moore JS: De Quervain's tenosynovitis: Stenosing tenosynovitis of the first dorsal compartment. J Occup Environ Med 39:990-1002,1997 in a general population. Occup Environ Med 54734-740,1997.

136. Nordstrom DL, Vierkant RA, DeStefano F, et al Risk factors for carpal tunnel syndrome Occup Med 7713-740, 1992.

137. Pelmear PL, Taylor W Hand-arm vibration syndrome: Clinical evaluation and prevention. J Occup Med 33:1144-1149,1991.

138. Pelmear PL, Taylor W Carpal tunnel syndrome and hand-arm vibration syndrome. Arch Neurol51:416-420,1994.

139. Piligian G, Herbert R, Hearns M, et al Evaluation and management of chronic workrelated musculoskeletal disorders of the distal upper extremity. Am J Ind Med 3775-93, 2000.

140. Reider B: The Orthopaedic Physical Examination. Philadelphia, WB Saunders, 1999.

141. Binder AI. Neck pain syndromes. Clinical Evidence. Search date December 2006. www.clinicalevidence.com/ceweb/conditions/msd/1103/1103_updates.jsp.

142. Binder AI. Cervical pain syndromes. In: Isenberg DA, Maddison PJ, Woo P, Glass DN, Breedveld FC, eds. Oxford textbook of rheumatology. 3rd ed. Oxford: Oxford Medical Publications, 2004:1185-95.

143. Vernon HT, Humphreys BK, Hagino CA. A systematic review of conservative treatments for acute neck pain not due to whiplash. J Manipulative Physiol Ther 2005;28:443-8.

144. Canadian Chiropractic Association, Canadian Federation of Chiropractic Regulatory Boards, Clinical Practice Guidelines Development Initiative, Guidelines Development Committee (GDC). Chiropractic clinical practice guideline: evidence-based treatment of adult neck pain not due to whiplash. J Can Chiropr Assoc 2005;49:158-209.

145. Aker PD, Gross AR, Goldsmith CH, Peloso P. Conservative management of mechanical neck pain: systematic overview and meta-analysis. BMJ 1996;313:1291-6.

146. Philadelphia Panel. Evidence-based clinical practice guidelines on selected rehabilitation interventions for neck pain. Phys Ther 2001;81:1701-17.

147. Sarig-Bahat H. Evidence for exercise therapy in mechanical neck disorders. Man Ther 2003;8:10-20.

148. Kay TM, Gross A, Goldsmith C, Santaguida PL, Hoving J, Brontfort G, et al, Cervical Overview Group. Exercises for mechanical neck disorders. Cochrane Database Syst Rev 2005;(3):CD004250.

149. Ylinen J, Takala E, Nykanen M, Hakknen A, Malkia E, Pohjolainen T, et al. Active neck muscle training in the treatment of chronic neck pain in women: a randomized controlled trial. JAMA 2003;289:2509-16.

150. Waling K, Sundelin G, Ahlgren C, Jarvholm B. Perceived pain before and after three exercise programs—a controlled clinical trial of women with work-related trapezius myalgia. Pain 2000;85:201-7.

151. Teichtahl AJ, McColl G. An approach to neck pain for the family physician. Aust Fam Physician. 2013;42(11):774-777.

152. Cohen SP. Epidemiology, diagnosis, and treatment of neck pain. Mayo Clin Proc. 2015;90(2):284-299.

153. Kumar PS, Kalpana RY. Clinico-radiological correlation in a cohort of cervical myelopathy patients. J Clin Diagn Res. 2015;9(1):TC01-TC07.

154. Hattou L, Morandi X, Le Reste PJ, Guillin R, Riffaud L, Hénaux PL. Dynamic cervical myelopathy in young adults. Eur Spine J. 2014;23(7):1515-1522.

155. Takahashi Y, Yasuhara T, Kumamoto S, et al. Laterality of cervical disc herniation. Eur Spine J. 2013;22(1):178-182.

156. Cheng X, Ni B, Liu Q, Chen J, Guan H, Guo Q. Clinical and radiological outcomes of spinal cord injury without radiologic evidence of trauma with cervical disc herniation. Arch Orthop Trauma Surg. 2013;133(2):193-198.

157. Ross DA, Ross MN. Diagnosis and treatment of C4 radiculopathy. Spine (Phila Pa 1976). 2016;41(23):1790-1794.

158. Jenkins TJ, Mai HT, Burgmeier RJ, Savage JW, Patel AA, Hsu WK. The triangle model of congenital cervical stenosis. Spine (Phila Pa 1976). 2016;41(5):E242-E247.

159. Morishita Y, Matsushita A, Maeda T, Ueta T, Naito M, Shiba K. Rapid progressive clinical deterioration of cervical spondylotic myelopathy. Spinal Cord. 2015;53(5):408-412.

160. Davies BM, McHugh M, Elgheriani A, et al. Reported outcome measures in degenerative cervical myelopathy: a systematic review. PLoS One. 2016;11(8):e0157263.

161. Eks̗i MS̗, Özcan Eks̗i EE, Yılmaz B, Toktas̗ ZO, Konya D. Cervical myelopathy due to single level disc herniation presenting as intramedullary mass lesion: what to do fi rst? J Craniovertebr Junction Spine. 2015;6(2):92-96.

162. Hoppenfeld S. Orthopaedic Neurology: A Diagnostic Guide to Neurologic Levels. 2nd ed. Philadelphia, PA: Wolters Kluwer; 2018.

163. Leichtle UG, Wünschel M, Socci M, Kurze C, Niemeyer T, Leichtle CI. Spine radiography in the evaluation of back and neck pain in an orthopaedic emergency clinic. J Back Musculoskelet Rehabil. 2015;28(1):43-48.

164. Bono CM, Ghiselli G, Gilbert TJ, et al. An evidence-based clinical guideline for the diagnosis and treatment of cervical radiculopathy from degenerative disorders. Spine J. 2011;11(1):64-72.

165. Cox J, DeGraauw C, Klein E. Pathological burst fracture in the cervical spine with negative red fl ags: a case report. J Can Chiropr Assoc. 2016;60(1):81-87.

166. McLaughlin N, Weil AG, Demers J, Shedid D. Klippel-Feil syndrome associated with a craniocervico-thoracic dermoid cyst. Surg Neurol Int. 2013;4(suppl 2):S61-S66.

167. Thoomes EJ. Effectiveness of manual therapy for cervical radiculopathy, a review. Chiropr Man Therap. 2016;24:45.

168. Manchikanti L, Falco FJ, Diwan S, Hirsch JA, Smith HS. Cervical radicular pain: the role of interlaminar and transforaminal epidural injections. Curr Pain Headache Rep. 2014;18(1):389.

169. Engquist M, Löfgren H, Öberg B, et al. A 5- to 8-year randomized study on the treatment of cervical radiculopathy: anterior cervical decompression and fusion plus physiotherapy versus physiotherapy alone. J Neurosurg Spine. 2017;26(1):19-27.

170. O'Reilly SC, Muir KR and Doherty M (1998) Knee pain and disability in the Nottingham community: association with poor health status and psychological distress. British Journal of Rheumatology 37: 870–873.

171. McAlindon TE, Cooper C, Kirwan JR and Dieppe PA (1992) Knee pain and disability in the community. British Journal of Rheumatology 31(3): 189–192.

172. Guccione AA, Felson DT, Anderson JJ et al (1994) The effects of specific medical conditions on the functional limitations of elders in the Framingham Study. American Journal of Public Health 84: 351–358.

173. Altman R, Asch E, Bloch D et al (1986) Development of criteria for the classification and reporting of osteoarthritis. Classification of osteoarthritis of the knee. Diagnostic and

Therapeutic Criteria Committee of the American Rheumatism Association. Arthritis and Rheumatism 29: 1039–1049.

174. van Saase JL, van Romunde LK, Cats A et al (1989) Epidemiology of osteoarthritis: Zoetermeer survey. Comparison of radiological osteoarthritis in a Dutch population with that in 10 other populations. Annals of the Rheumatic Diseases 48: 271–280.

175. Oliveria SA, Felson DT, Reed JI et al (1995) Incidence of symptomatic hand, hip, and knee osteoarthritis among patients in a health maintenance organization. Arthritis and Rheumatism 38: 1134–1141.

176. Kosorok MR, Omenn GS, Diehr P et al (1992) Restricted activity days among older adults. American Journal of Public Health 82: 1263–1267.

177. Kramer JS, Yelin EH and Epstein WV (1983) Social and economic impacts of four musculoskeletal conditions. A study using national community-based data. Arthritis and Rheumatism 26: 901–907.

178. The Incidence and Prevalence Database for Procedures (1995) The Incidence and Prevalence Database for Procedures. Sunnyvale, CA: Timely Data Resources.

179. Lawrence JS, De Graaj R and Laine VAI (1962) The Epidemiology of Chronic Rheumatism. Oxford: Blackwell.

180. Altman RD, Hochberg M, Murphy WA Jr et al (1995) Atlas of individual radiographic features in osteoarthritis. Osteoarthritis and Cartilage 3 (supplement A): 3–70.

181. Felson DT, McAlindon TE, Anderson JJ et al (1997) Defining radiographic osteoarthritis for the whole knee. Osteoarthritis and Cartilage 5: 241–250.

182. Carlesso LC, Gross AR, MacDermid JC, Walton DM, Santaguida PL. Pharmacological, psychological, and patient education interventions for patients with neck pain: results of an international survey. J Back Musculoskelet Rehabil. 2015;28(3):561-573.

183. Oral A, Sindel D, Ketenci A. Evidence-based physical medicine and rehabilitation strategies for patients with cervical radiculopathy due to disc herniation. Turk J Phys Med Rehab. 2014;60:47-53.

184. Salo P, Ylo"nen-Ka"yra" N, Ha"kkinen A, Kautiainen H, Ma"lkia" E, Ylinen J. Effects of long-term home-based exercise on health-related quality of life in patients with chronic neck pain: a randomized study with a 1-year follow-up. Disabil Rehabil 2012;34:1971-7.

185. Ha"kkinen A, Kautiainen H, Hannonen P, Ylinen J. Strength training and stretching versus stretching only in the treatment of patients with chronic neck pain: a randomized one-year follow-up study. Clin Rehabil 2008;22:592-600.

186. Falla D, Jull G, Hodges P, Vicenzino B. An endurance-strength training regime is effective in reducing myoelectric manifiestations of cervical flexor muscle fatigue in females with chronic neck pain. Clin Neurophysiol 2006;117:828-37.

187. Evans R, Bronfort G, Schulz C, et al. Supervised exercise with and without spinal manipulation performs similarly and better than home exercise for chronic neck pain: a randomized controlled trial. Spine (Phila Pa 1976) 2012;37:903-14.

Chapter 4:

Workplace Prevention And Management Strategies

By decreasing or removing external burdens, altering organisational factors, changing the social environment, enhancing personal stress-coping abilities, and corresponding the physical demands of the job to the employee's physical capabilities, both primary and secondary actions can avoid negative outcomes. According to the literature, some of these strategies are more effective than others. Some interventions had not yet undergone thorough evaluation [1,2].

Internal stresses on tissues as well as other anatomical structures are produced by the body's response to external stressors in the workplace. The movements and pressures acting upon the individual, particularly vibration and heat exposures, must be identified and quantified prior to any interventions that aim to reduce or eliminate exposure to external loads. It is frequently necessary to do a thorough analysis of the task to assess these physical exposures and their unique characteristics [3]. The causes for these loads are identified when particular psychological factors are discovered. Depending on how they contribute to the identified pressures, workplace redesign may involve changes to the tools, equipment, workplaces, materials dealing with tasks, working techniques, work processes, and overall work environment. This strategy for reducing injuries is the foundation of the majority of intervention literature [4].

Job content and organisation features, as well as the temporal and financial components of the work and task, make up the wide category of work organisational factors. The variety of tasks and processes that go into creating a job description constitute its content. The contact with external loads related to the usage of tools and equipment is directly impacted by these criteria [5]. Requirements to handle certain products, operate equipment, or work in potentially hazardous environments are examples of additional job content. By directly changing the job requirements, modifications to the job content can minimise or completely remove exposure to physical stress. Examples include dividing up a worker's duties or automating the removal of a certain duty [6].

The managerial structure of the company and the degree of employee autonomy are both described by organisational features. These elements may have an impact on how employees feel about their jobs or how much physical stress they experience. Relationships between coworkers and managers may also affect how much physical stress is exposed. For instance, when workers formally help one another, physical pressures within an atmosphere of cooperation are frequently lessened. Temporal characteristics of work include shift work, the number of hours till the deadline, job rotation, and the frequency and length of a particular task. For instance, performing boring, repetitive work continuously has been linked to both physical and mental stress [4,5].

Last but not least, a company's financial planning, attention toward human resource management, and employees' individual awareness have an impact on physical exposure. For instance, working longer hours and overtime might prolong daily exposure to musculoskeletal stresses. Compensation incentives may also have an impact on the quantity, frequency, and length of labour as well as discourage taking pauses for relaxation [6].

Principles of ergonomics

Most intervention material is based on the use of ergonomic concepts. The investigation of work, particularly workplace modifications to ensure compatibility between the worker, the task, and the workplace, is known as ergonomics. Researchers and practitioners in a variety of fields, such as medicine, epidemiology, psychology, industrial engineering, and other health-related, technical/engineering, and behavioural disciplines, are involved in the field of ergonomics. These professionals represent the variety of factors that influence workplace safety and productivity [7].

The procedure for applying ergonomics to intervention follows the scientific method: data is collected and analysed (for example, through local or wide surveillance and analysis for jobs); hypotheses are created (for example, particular engineering controls are suggested to address specific variables or circumstances for the physical workplace as well as job features). Managerial measures are proposed to address the features of the organisation and management. Recent research suggests that workplace musculoskeletal illnesses and the accompanying impairment are the results of a complex interaction between workplace, individual, and social psychosocial elements as well as medical, social, organisational, and biomechanical aspects [8]. The ergonomics treatment within the workplace offers a growing body of knowledge and a developing set of interventions, as is true for most scientific fields of study. To enable the efficient management as well as prevention of such complex disorders, further development for innovative models is required. The practise of ergonomics depends on a process that assesses novel treatments, adapts interventions to particular situations where they are currently determined to be beneficial, and keeps evaluating the efficacy of these interventions the light of shifting workplace and worker conditions [9]. Therefore, it is neither practicable nor desirable to suggest general treatments that are anticipated to fit every sector, job, or worker, nor "once for all" interventions whose success does not need to be continuously evaluated. Instead, it is both possible and desirable to promote the use of interventions that have so far been found to be effective and promising, as well as to promote collaboration and information sharing among researchers, practitioners, as well as employees/managers in business/labor, politics, and academia. Intervention practice and research both heavily rely on surveillance and job analysis [8,9].

Surveillance

In order to describe and monitor work-related musculoskeletal illnesses and assess the efficacy of the programme, surveillance is the continual, systematic gathering, analysis, and comprehension of wellness and exposure information. As a kind of surveillance, employees may be surveyed via questionnaire or physical examination (active surveillance), or existing medical records and worker compensation records may be analysed (passive surveillance) [10]. Figure 19 and Figure 20 show the ergonomic specifications to be maintained while working in sitting and standing positions, respectively.

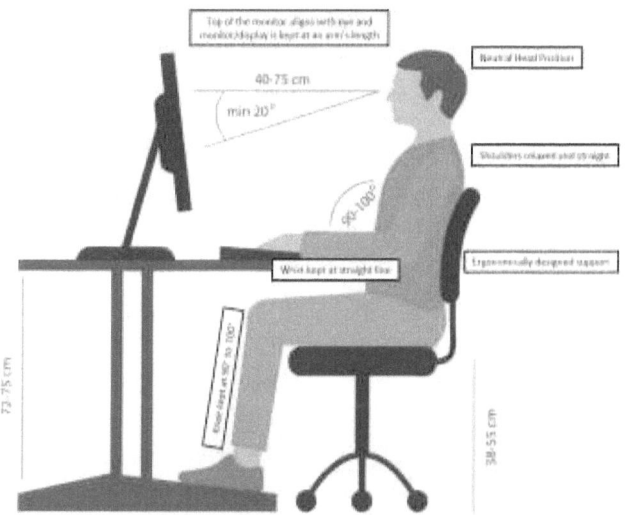

Figure 19: Typical guidelines for maintaining a correct posture while working on desktop

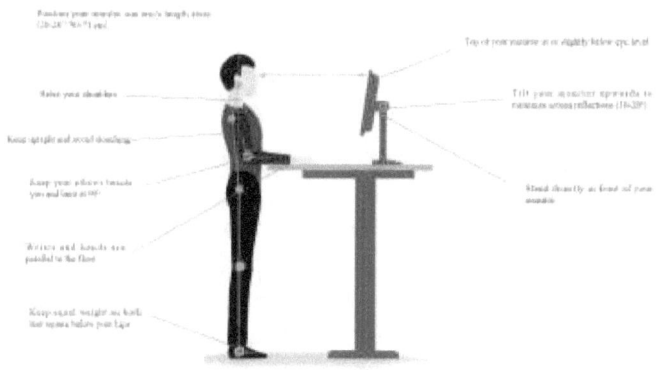

Figure 20: Typical guidelines for maintaining a correct posture while standing and performing works on the table

Although analysing information already in existence is typically less expensive, it can be challenging to determine how reliable the data is. Although it is uncertain if the added expense of an active monitoring system will discourage the normal use of such systems, standardised questionnaires and physical tests may be as sensitive as the use of exceptionally complete current occupational medical records. In the context of cooperative labor-management ergonomics programmes, symptom questionnaires, and checklist-based hazard surveillance were practical as well as more sensitive to ergonomic issues than existent sources of information [11].

Surveillance systems are important tools for gathering data on worker characteristics (individual factors) that might interact with workplace variables to exacerbate or ameliorate musculoskeletal illnesses or alter the effectiveness of therapies. Systems of surveillance may also be employed to assess the efficacy of initiatives. Additionally, monitoring systems (such as employee surveys, absentee as well as turnover analysis, job analysis, work flow evaluation, and productivity studies) can be used to gather data that supports other analytical procedures in defining pertinent characteristics of tasks, jobs, employee happiness, as well as organisational culture. When the economy is changing quickly and there may not be enough resources for prevention, surveillance is more crucial [12].

A thorough examination of risk variables is conducted after an employment methods analysis, which is based on a time-and-motion study to ascertain the job's work content. In order to analyse work procedures, each task's work content is broken down into a number of phases or components, and each component's risk factors are identified [12]. After determining the primary physical stressors, ergonomic solutions can be used to reduce risk factor exposure. Engineering controls, administrative and production controls, and personal modifiers are common categories for such interventions. Although risk variables are widely mentioned in the literature, safe exposure limits for each one separately as well as when combined have not yet been established [13]. The existence of a hazard does not always indicate that the person performing the task is at an elevated risk of harm or that the expense of making ergonomic adjustments is justified. When risk indicators are present and people who do that work have a history of having musculoskeletal problems, the risk could be deemed overly high, and ergonomic treatments may be cost-effective. Regardless of the past, it is frequently advisable to change because work changes are frequently affordable and injuries are frequently quite expensive. This is especially true when occupations are first conceived and established [14].

Developing Effective Ergonomic Programs

Both industrialised (developed) nations and industrially developing countries (IDCs) must work to enhance occupational health by reducing the prevalence of musculoskeletal diseases (MSDs). Musculoskeletal illnesses are currently responsible for 40% of occupational and work-related health expenses worldwide, thus both DCs and IDCs should be concerned. The majority of the working population in IDCs is engaged in agricultural trades, so efforts to implement ergonomics programmes within IDCs have primarily concentrated on large-scale industries. Ergonomic interventions, therefore, must be adaptable enough to move above the factory environment towards rural villages. This calls for a low-cost, simple-to-understand programming procedure that is considerate of the social, cultural, and political concerns of a particular people [15].

Intervention methods with an emphasis on prevention should be used in an ergonomics programme. Particularly in occupations where workers are exposed to a high level of incidence of occupational risk factors, ergonomic treatments have proved beneficial in lowering the occurrence of MSDs to over 50%. Agriculture, construction, mining, fishing, and logging are recognised hazardous occupations in IDCs with significant physical demands [16]. The worker must be actively involved in initiatives that also limit their exposure to this stressor and change the organisational culture. There is a higher chance that ergonomic treatments including the worker may lessen musculoskeletal issues. Participatory ergonomics is cited as a key strategy for reducing MSDs and launching an ergonomics programme in recent recommendations to the United States National Institute for Occupational Health and Safety (NIOSH), European Agency over Safety as well as Health at Work (EASHW), and General Accounting Office (GAO) [17].

The GAO study emphasises the factors that make ergonomics programmes successful. Five businesses were examined, and the synopsis highlights a core group of six factors: (1) commitment from management, (2) staff engagement, (3) recognising problem jobs, (4) creation of solutions (controls) over problem jobs, (5) education and training for employees, or (6) suitable medical management. The use of these components has decreased the number of accidents and illnesses and also the expense of worker compensation. Additionally, surveys indicated increased worker satisfaction, output, and product quality [18].

The GAO goes on to suggest that federal and state-run OSHA programmes use a similar strategy when creating a framework for worksite ergonomic programmes that emphasises the necessity of creating and putting into place flexible site-specific attempts that efficiently address hazards. The NIOSH paper suggests concentrating on reducing MSDs at work [19]. The following seven actions are provided in this book to help you detect, treat, and prevent MSDs: identifying and meeting training needs, gathering and analysing data to define the nature and extent of ergonomics concerns, developing control solutions, creating health care management, determining whether there are musculoskeletal problems in the workplace, developing roles over managers and employees in an ergonomic programme, recognising and meeting training needs, developing an ergonomics programme that is proactive. The GAO recommendations are supplemented by NIOSH with the addition of two crucial criteria: data collection and analysis, as well as a focus on developing proactive programmes [20].

Risk assessment, health monitoring, information for staff, training, ergonomic workplaces, and fatigue prevention are all included in the EASHW report's definition of the scope for preventing work-related upper limb diseases. approaches for assessing exposure and risk are proposed while acknowledging that these approaches frequently conflict with the reality of field use. The adoption of an integrated ergonomic intervention that concentrates on the entire workplace and work system is also emphasized in the paper. Participatory ergonomics may be able to help with the creation of this comprehensive strategy [21].

Participatory ergonomics

Both organisational management and researchers have engaged in a great deal of "trial and error" while implementing participatory programmes inside the workplace. The potential advantages of workplace engagement are supported by academic research and theory. Benefits include improved performance and worker health, higher employee motivation and job satisfaction, a decrease in work-related musculoskeletal disorders (WRMDs), quicker organisational and technological change implementation, and more thorough ergonomics problem diagnosis and solution development [22]. A theoretical framework along with design guidelines that address the implementation of participatory programmes are nonetheless absent. The question "why participation?" is therefore easily answered, but "how are effective participatory programmes achieved?" is less clear. We may have a reason to pursue participatory ergonomics as a practise based on prior theories and studies that support its value, but there is little guidance on how to go about it in order to prevent WRMDs over the long term, improve quality of working life (QWL), and increase organisational effectiveness [23].

One intervention technique that can address both ergonomic and psychological risk factors within the workplace is participatory ergonomics. This approach involves "end-users" of ergonomics actively participating in the discovery and evaluation of ergonomics hazards as well as the creation and use of ergonomics solutions. In order to enhance the psychosocial elements of work and hence lower the chance of developing WRMDs, the participatory ergonomic method incorporates training for the workforce, improved information interchange, and employee engagement in decision-making [24].

'Selective' and 'continuous improvement' involvement are crucially dissimilar, according to Zink (1996). Utilising participatory techniques for certain organisational tasks, such as the adoption of new technology, is known as selective participation. However, participation in continuous improvement refers to the application of participatory techniques in an effort to accomplish continuous improvement inside an organization. Both forms of engagement are beneficial and do not conflict with one another. Participation in continuous improvement, however, covers the greater ground and is related to the ideas of organizational learning and organizational culture. The 'in-house' participatory ergonomic program implementation procedure described here is centered on this kind of engagement [25].

The organizational culture must change for the adoption of continuous improvement participation. Participation is a way of life at work rather than being contained in a single or small number of particular initiatives. Implementing an 'in-house' participatory ergonomics program involves implementing ergonomics as well as ergonomic ideas, training and education, individual as well as group learning, and the provision of resources, with the ultimate goal of enabling organizational members to become competent in resolving work-related issues as well as planning for growth and development on their own. Through engagement that spreads across the organization over time, the 'in-house' participatory ergonomics program enables continual development [26].

The benefits of adopting a continuous improvement strategy for participation ought to be obvious. It takes a comprehensive approach towards participation, allowing for results that go beyond those that are frequently associated with gains in workplace engagement (such as higher employee motivation or a more open-minded attitude towards change). Creating a feeling of community at work, fostering ongoing learning and development among organizational members, and continuously improving working conditions, work organization, job design, and interpersonal communication are further benefits [27].

Ergonomics in industries

Human factors and ergonomics Engineering is concerned with using knowledge of human behaviour, capabilities, and limits to create systems, devices, instruments, tasks/jobs, settings, etc. for human usage that is efficient, safe, and effective. an industrial. Industry includes a complex system of people, machines, environments, and organizations for efficiency and productivity. The administration of this system should guarantee the best possible performance of the system's components. The work should be adapted to the person performing it, not the other way around [28].

The need to increase manufacturing sectors' efficiency, security, and quality is becoming more and more important. These sectors have a number of characteristics, including bad workplace design, poorly organised occupations, an unfavourable work environment, subpar human-machine system design, and inadequate management strategies. They cause job risks, poor worker health, injuries from mechanical equipment, and disabilities, which in turn lower worker productivity, lower the calibre of the produced goods, and raise costs [29]. Therefore, achieving the goals of the industrial sectors would be incredibly challenging without giving ergonomics the right consideration. A balance among worker characteristics and job demands may be achieved via the successful integration of ergonomics into work system design. This may increase employee productivity while also ensuring their safety, physical and emotional health, and workplace happiness [30].

Ergonomics research has also resulted in data and recommendations for industrial use. It is common knowledge that machinery, workstations, and facilities should be designed ergonomically. In the industrial industry, however, it has still a low degree of acceptability and little use. The enhancement of machines and equipment alone is typically the primary objective of work system design. The whole work system is given either little or no thought. As a result, poorly designed work processes are widespread in the industrial sector. The workforce suffers from inefficiency and suffering when ergonomic principles are ignored. Low productivity, poor job quality, and physical and mental stress can all result from an ergonomically unsound workplace [31].

The application of ergonomics has helped to lower workplace injuries. Although the current focus is on musculoskeletal diseases, ergonomics has historically been utilised to boost productivity and efficiency. The fundamental ideas of ergonomics may be applied to increase workplace efficiency and safety. By combining ergonomics and productivity, workstations may be created to maximise performance and cut expenses. Productivity was shown to increase dramatically when ergonomics were included in industrial work designs [32]. It is thought that poor ergonomics in the industrial sector is to blame for occupational health risks, a lack of safety, and decreased worker quality and efficiency. Insufficient ergonomics knowledge, training, and resources are probably to blame for the poor adoption and use of ergonomics [33].

Ergonomic programs in dentistry

Dental workers frequently can't avoid PSPs, or extended static postures. More than half of the body's muscles are clenched statically even in the best sitting positions, and the vertebral joints barely move. This might lead to harmful physiological alterations (microchanges) that can cause musculoskeletal diseases, or MSDs, or back, neck, or shoulder discomfort (macrochanges) [33,34]. These postural and positional issues, as well as the ensuing harmful physiological changes—muscle imbalances, stiff joints, muscle necrosis, and spinal disc degeneration—must be addressed through prevention tactics and ergonomic procedures in order to effectively avoid injuries in dentistry [34].

Post-Awareness Practises

Keep your low back curvature. According to research, keeping the lumbar lordosis when sitting might lessen or even eliminate low back discomfort. The low back curvature can be preserved by implementing the following habits [35,36]. To accentuate the low back curvature, tilt the seat five to fifteen degrees forward. This will raise the hips over the knees and make a hip angle bigger than 90 degrees, which could enable you to position yourself closer to the patient. An ergonomic wedge-shaped cushion may be installed into chairs without a tilt function [34-36].

Sit next to the patient and, if feasible, place your knees beneath the patient's chair. Tilting the chair and employing patient chairs with headrests and thin upper backs can help with this. This configuration may produce arm abduction or shoulder elevation in some operators. In these circumstances, a new working posture ought to be taken [37,38].

Use an operator stool with a saddle-style seat to encourage the low back's natural curvature by making the hip angle around 130 degrees. In situations when the patient seats feature thick backs and headrests, using this sort of stool could enable you to be closer to the patient [36-37].

Put the feet firmly onto the floor to equally distribute your weight and raise the chair so that the hips are just above the knees. The thighs' backs shouldn't be compressed by the chair's forward edge. By moving the lumbar support forward to make touch with the floor, make use of the chair's lumbar support as much as feasible. By tightening the transverse abdominal muscles, you may stabilise the low back curvature. In order to do it while sitting, maintain a tiny curvature in the back area, sit tall, inhale, and bring the navel towards the floor without allowing the curve to flatten. Maintaining a contraction during one breath cycle while continuing to breathe [38,39].

Magnification is used. Magnification systems that are chosen, adjusted and used correctly have been linked to reduced neck and lower back discomfort as they enable operators to keep more wholesome postures. When choosing and utilising a magnification system, bear the following in mind [38].

There are operational flip-up or through-the-lens telescopes and loupes available. You should be able to maintain a neck flexion of no more than 20 degrees thanks to the descent angle of the scopes [37,38]. Neck discomfort has been linked to positions when the neck is flexed more than 20 degrees during work. To find out which functioning telescope type best fits your demands and your personality, you should test out a few different ones. The elbows should be near the sides and the shoulders should be relaxed when working at this distance [39].

You can view working field detail with a magnification of 2 that is about equivalent to what you would see while crouching over the patient sans scopes. Greater than 2-magnification results in improved clarity of vision but a reduced field of view. Operating microscopes are built to encourage the most neutral postures and offer the maximum magnification of all systems that are now available [38-40].

Correctly adjust the operator's chair. Chaffin and colleagues claim that the days of treating postural issues caused by prolonged sitting at work by merely providing a chair are past. To get the most ergonomic benefits, operators must understand how to alter the characteristics of their seats [41]. First, adjust the seat. Operators frequently make the error of situating patients first, and then changing their seats to fit them. When working with clients who are old or handicapped, accommodations can be made. Place the buttocks firmly against the chair's back [41,42]. The sides of the knees shouldn't be in contact with the seat edge. You may be tempted to lean over the edge of a seat if it is too deep. Place feet flat on the ground and raise the seat height until thighs are softly sloping down and feet are still flat on the ground [40-42]. This makes it easier for you to put your knees beneath the patient and keeps the low back curvature in place. Adjust the backrest so that the lumbar support sits comfortably within the lower back's natural lumbar curvature. The lumbar support should then be angled forward to make reaching the lower back easier. Tilt the seat five to fifteen degrees forward. Start off using the seat tilt mechanism with a little tilt and then gradually raise it until you feel comfortable. Adjust armrests to support elbows while maintaining a neutral shoulder position, which will lessen neck and shoulder pain and strain [42,43].

Positioning methods

Avoid being still. Lehto and colleagues assert that the idea of a single proper work position may be physically false since the human body might have been built for movement and constantly shifting postures. Sitting and standing should be alternated. Alternating between the two positions allows one set of muscles to relax while the effort is transferred to another pair of muscles since standing and sitting engage distinct muscle groups. The feet should be moved. One set of low back muscles' burden can be shifted to another by making little adjustments to one's foot position, allowing nutrients to be replenished into the overworked tissues. Place the patients in the right height positions. a typical error made by dentists [44].

Implementing Injury Prevention Measures

The application of professional guidance

In professional settings, recommendations for modifications to work processes, workplace culture, and individual work practises being frequently included in ergonomics and injury prevention advice. Even when deliberately sought out, this advise might not be properly followed or might just be disregarded. This is made worse by the lack of regular review of the use and efficacy of the supplied recommendations by ergonomics experts [45]. The lack of evaluation to examine the application of ergonomics advice offered by qualified ergonomics consultants has primarily been attributed to client/company disinterest because of associated costs, but it has also in part been attributed to the consultants' beliefs that request over evaluation could suggest a lack of confidence in the efficacy of the interventions they had suggested. The failure to put recommendations into practise may be due to a variety of factors, such as cost, efficacy, the consultant's lack of comprehension of the company's goals, or the company's lack of "desire" to make changes. These elements imply that consultants should structure their recommendations to increase their likelihood of being adopted [46].

Methods for changing behaviour

Advice on injury prevention frequently suggests modifying the workplace, organisational structures, and individual work habits. A shift in conduct is a necessary component of such transformations. According to the principles of behaviour modification, several strategies have been put forth to enhance the adoption and efficacy of ergonomics recommendations. Prochaska and DiClemente's Stage of Modification (SOC) paradigm, which assigns respondents to one of five phases based on their willingness to change using a brief sequence of closed questions, has been the approach of behaviour modification that has been used in workplace settings the most frequently [47,48].

1. Pre-contemplation (not knowing or not caring about job risks)

2. Contemplation (thinking about change but hesitating to take action)

3. Planning (to alter the very near future)

4. Take action (make modifications during the last six months)

5. Maintenance (changes were made, and efforts are being made to consolidate gains and prevent relapse)

Then, in order to increase receptivity, advice is adapted in accordance with the stage of the shift. For instance, people who are in the earlier stages are going to benefit from knowledge about the risks and hazards associated with their current behaviour as well as actions, which could promote progression onto later stages, while those in the later phases will benefit to practical information regarding how to make, or maintain change [49].

The SOC strategy has been assessed by tracking post-intervention progress through the several phases of change, believing that individuals in later stages become more "risk aware" and hence engage in less risky activity. Changes in self-reported body part discomfort and safety culture have also been used as additional metrics to gauge success [50].

Despite roughly 100 million work-related injuries happening worldwide each year, they continue to put a significant strain on both employees and businesses. Musculoskeletal disorders (MSD), commonly referred to are ergonomic injuries, are still common, frequently cause a significant burden of disability, and have high related costs. The US Bureau of Labour Statistics (BLS) estimated that there were >2.8 million nonfatal occupational injury cases in private industries in 2011, and that >50% of these instances required days off work, job transfers, or work restrictions [47]. In 2011, 33% of all illnesses and accidents at work that required time off were MSDs. Occupational disorders continue to be a significant burden on society in general as well as workplaces in particular due to lost productivity, decreased performance, lost-time claims, as well as medical costs among those impacted within the short term as well as potential effects in turnover, job engagement, as well as morale over time. This is true even though the incidence rate and number of occupational injuries with work-related MSD have declined in recent years [45].

The risk of occupational injury and MSD is enhanced by a variety of physical and psychological exposures, work organisational characteristics, and individual variables (including anthropometrics that body mass index, illness status, sex, employment tenure, and hours worked). Consequently, even for employees performing the same job responsibilities, individual worker risk might vary significantly. This well-known complex nature of causation makes it challenging to research how ergonomic improvements affect injury outcomes [48,49].

Workers in a wide variety of jobs are affected by physical workplace exposures associated with duties, the working setting, and the use of equipment and materials. These exposures are significantly linked to the risk of injury and there is some evidence of an exposure-response relationship. Forceful manual handling, uncomfortable neck, back, and lower extremity positions, repetitive movements, contact stress, segmental and whole-body vibration, and exposure to severe temperatures are only a few examples of these exposures. According to an up-to-date assessment of physical occupational hazards in the US workforce, 10% of workers are exposed to squeezed work spaces which necessitate the adoption of awkward postures on a daily basis, 2.7% are exposed for whole body vibration, and 27% spend more than half their workdays bending or twisting [50].

A number of workplace ergonomic treatments were developed to tackle ergonomic hazards without varying degrees of reported effectiveness utilising an array of outcome measures in recognition of the importance of these physical exposures at work to injury and MSD risk. A comprehensive ergonomic approach to danger reduction with active worker involvement can be a successful way to lower the risk of damage from workplace exposures [51]. However, there is conflicting evidence regarding how these participatory ergonomics affect various outcomes. Some studies indicate a positive impact on employee satisfaction with work and morale but fail to demonstrate any impact on injury risk, while other studies indicate a decrease in injury incidence, severity, or cost. Nevertheless, several nations now mandate that businesses manage injury risk while involving employees who are most at risk in the procedure [52].

There are no explicit ergonomic regulation standards in the US, despite the fact that US workers are exposed to a high amount of ergonomic risks and that workplace modifications to better fit workers can reduce the risk of harm through participatory ergonomics along with other methods [52].

Although there are voluntary ergonomics standards for many industries, the current study indicates that without the realistic prospect of enforcement, such initiatives may not accomplish much to motivate the businesses that most need to improve [53].

A multinational manufacturer of aluminium and associated products with operations in the US and other countries launched a targeted, internal company-wide initiative to identify and manage ergonomic risks in manufacturing and upkeep tasks across all active sites. A business directive that each operating plant must (i) identify the ten work tasks that need ergonomic improvement the most and (ii) implement control for a minimum of half of the aforementioned issue jobs by the end of 2003 marked the beginning of the project. This programme acted as a prelude to the company's implementation of an obligatory ergonomics standard at the end of 2001, which was largely based on the OSHA ergonomics regulation that had previously been temporarily released before being withdrawn. In order to identify all ergonomic risks, save them to the company's database of ergonomic hazards, and put suitable controls in place for half of these hazards by the end of 2006, factories were expected to start performing work task-oriented quantitative ergonomic risk evaluations in 2004. Its ergonomic hazards database has been revised to reflect new hazard controls (HC) when they were put into place [54].

Ergonomic hazard identification and control implementation on musculoskeletal disorder and injury risk

With roughly 100 million work-related injuries happening worldwide each year (1), they continue to put a significant strain on both employees and businesses. Musculoskeletal disorders (MSD), frequently referred to are ergonomic injuries, are still common and can cause significant disability and high related expenses. The US Bureau of Labour Statistics (BLS) estimated that there were >2.8 million nonfatal occupational injury cases in private businesses in 2011; >50% of these instances required days off work, job transfers, or work restrictions. In 2011, 33% of all occupational illnesses and injuries necessitating time off work were MSD [55]. These occupational disorders continue to be a significant burden on society in general as well as workplaces in particular, despite a recent decline in both the incidence rate as well as the number of occupational injuries and work-related MSDs). This is due to lost productivity, decreased performance, lost-time claims, as well as medical costs between affected workers in the short term, as well as potential long-term effects on turnover, job engagement, as well as morale. The risk of occupational injury and MSD is raised by a variety of physical and psychological exposures, work organisational characteristics, and individual variables (like anthropometrics, body mass index, illness status, sex, employment tenure, and hours worked) [56].

Consequently, even for employees performing the same job responsibilities, individual worker risk might vary significantly. This well-known complex nature of causation makes it challenging to research how ergonomic improvements affect injury outcomes. Workers in a wide variety of jobs are affected by physical workplace exposures associated with duties, the working setting, and the use of equipment and materials. These exposures are significantly linked to the risk of injury and there is some evidence of an exposure-response relationship [57].

Forceful manual handling, uncomfortable neck, back, and lower extremity positions, repetitive movements, contact stress, segmental and whole-body vibration, and exposure to severe temperatures are only a few examples of these exposures.A number of workplace ergonomic treatments are being implemented to tackle ergonomic hazards with varying degrees of reported effectiveness utilising a range of outcome measures in recognition of the importance of these physical exposures at work to injury and MSD risk. Using a diversified ergonomic strategy to reduce risk and including workers actively in the process helps reduce the risk of injuries from occupational exposures [58].

There are no specific ergonomic regulatory requirements in the US, despite the fact that US workers are exposed to a high amount of ergonomic risks and that workplace modifications that better meet workers can reduce the risk of injury via participatory ergonomics as well as other methods. Although there are voluntary ergonomics recommendations for many industries, new research indicates that without the realistic prospect of enforcement, such initiatives may not accomplish much to motivate the employers who most need to improve to take action [59].

4.3 Training and Education for Employees and Employers

The workplace is a complicated system with many interrelated elements that affect the worker, including environmental, physical, psychological, organisational, and individual aspects. The International Ergonomics Association (IEA) defines ergonomics as "the scientific discipline concerned with understanding the interactions among humans as well as other elements of a system in order to optimise human well-being as well as overall system performance" (International Ergonomics Association, 2019). Ergonomics and wellness promotion interventions, particularly those provided online, have become crucial to preventing the occurrence for these health issues due to the rapid increase within computers along with desk-based work and the associated effects of prolonged sitting as well as prolonged computer screen seeing in health outcomes like musculoskeletal conditions (MSDs), eye strain, heart disease, work strain, and psychological distress [60].

The cornerstones of ergonomic interventions are training and education. Despite the fact that there is no single, widely accepted definition for office ergonomics training, it is generally agreed upon that it should include activities that help workers detect risk factors over work-related MSDs, choose and use the right tools and practises, and correctly adjust their workstations so they are user-friendly and promote a pleasant place to work. Office ergonomics education and training programmes have had varying degrees of success. While improvements in knowledge, reduced musculoskeletal pain, adopting healthy behaviours, and improved performance have all been noted, non-statistically influences on these outcomes are also noted [61]. Furthermore, it has been noted that the quality of the evidence resulting from ergonomics educational initiatives is poor. When paired with additional tactics like workstation redesign and participatory ergonomics interventions, ergonomics training proved most successful. Additionally, from the viewpoint of instructional design, the manner ergonomics training was produced and the usage using instructional system development models, theories of learning, and end-user engagement for successful training materials might have an impact on the training's efficacy. In order to address how office workers interact with other system components, ergonomics training programmes should use a holistic approach to content development that takes into account the physical, organisational, or cognitive realms (International Ergonomic Association, 2019). Programmes for workplace education and training in ergonomics have been delivered using a variety of techniques [62].

These techniques include face-to-face one-on-one instruction or group-based delivery like workshops, technology-based learning (PC, cellphones, tablets) via interactive multimedia and web-based programmes, or a hybrid of the two. Online (virtual/e-learning) tools are now an efficient technique to monitor and enhance people's health as a result of technological advancements and broad access to the Internet and mobile devices. Virtual refers to technologies that use a computer along with other electronic devices but do not require people to physically travel anywhere, according to the Cambridge Dictionary (2020) [62].

Online education is becoming more and more common, and it has shown to be a successful method of professional development in a variety of fields, including higher education, healthcare (for example, for health professionals), and business and administration (for example, for office employees). Widespread accessibility, individualised education, and frequent material updates are just a few of the possible benefits of online learning over conventional training techniques. In the United States, 39% of organisations' formal learning hours were spent using technology-based learning in 2012. This involves e-learning, online learning, and mobile learning [63]. Online learning is now the most popular way to conduct workplace training, according to more current statistics by the Australian Bureau for Statistics (2022), which indicated that it climbed from 19% in 2016–17 to 55% in 2020–21. Virtual/e-learning has been regarded as the most appropriate delivery method for training programmes since it allows for flexibility in terms of time and place as well as the ability for instruction personalization. Due to the COVID-19 pandemic's increased share of office labour occurring at home, the capacity to learn and conduct self-evaluation remotely is of special importance [64].

There isn't a synthesis of data regarding the types of programmes that are available, their content, and the accessibility, feasibility, acceptability, and users' satisfaction with these training programmes, according to a preliminary and exploratory search of the literature for virtual and e-learning ergonomics training programmes for office workers. These aspects of training programme design have been recognised as crucial elements in the success if the e-learning process [65]. Researchers have also placed a strong emphasis on the pedagogical components of producing e-learning, including the application of instructional design theories and models to pinpoint users' individual requirements and produce the desired results (such as information acquisition, skill development, or behaviour modification). It's probable that there are ergonomics training courses offered by organisations like health and safety at work authorities outside of the realm of standard scientific publications. In order to help industries satisfy their legal obligations to lower the risk for workplace injuries and protect employee safety and health, these agencies offer services and resources [66]. We do not, however, know if local, national, and international Occupational Health and Safety (OHS) agencies and organisations provide office workers and workplaces with online training programmes that are effective and have the appropriate material. Future development of these programmes will benefit by finding any current online training programmes in the literature that has been peer-reviewed or offered by OHS authorities and describing their content, usability, and functioning aspects [67].

Return to Work Programs and Accommodations

High absence rates owing to prevalent mental (e.g., anxiety, melancholy) and musculoskeletal illnesses (CMDs and MSDs) remain despite a variety of policies, recommendations, and best practices implemented by employers and governments to decrease days missed to sickness absence. On the one hand, CMDs are the most prevalent mental health issues—including stress, anxiety, and depression—that are reported. According to the Health and Safety Executive (HSE), these frequently result from stressful life events or experiences that affect a person's capacity to perform at work, at home, or in a mix of both [38]. On the contrary, MSDs is a condition that affects the joints, muscles, bones, and nearby connective tissues. It is often described by discomfort (which is frequently chronic), restrictions in range of motion, and a lack of dexterity, which makes it harder for patients to work and engage in society. The need to identify the most efficient means of assisting sick-listed workers to return to the workforce (RTW) is strengthened by the fact that these diseases may become chronic with high rates of recurrence, placing people at a higher risk of early withdrawal from the labour force and at a larger risk of being excluded. 1.8 million UK employees experienced work-related sickness in January 2022

[39].914,000 of those 1.8 million employees missed work due to CMDs, while 477,000 did so due to MSDs. These conditions have an annual considerable increase in absenteeism rates, which may indicate a lack of initiatives for helping people return to work. We are concentrating particularly on CMDs and MSDs throughout our study because of this. We think that the results of this study will help companies and the government cut down on absence rates and expenses [40].

RTW is crucial because employment offers benefits including self-esteem, social connections, and financial security to workers. There are conflicts between what workers need to reintegrate into the workforce and what companies require for a quick return to work, though. Additionally, because of the health and financial advantages of working, sick-listed workers constitute the least powerful players yet would benefit the most from a successful RTW. Understanding workplace factors that affect sustainable RTW is of utmost importance, particularly when these factors are a result of a larger systemic/organizational issue, given the effect of the COVID-19 pandemic on risk factors and the incidence of MSDs as well as CMDs, such as those related to remote working and using inappropriate equipment [41].

Early RTW speeds up the recovery process from illness, but for workers who have been sick-listed with CMDs including MSDs, the process of return to work is complicated, including many interrelated considerations and the collaboration of several stakeholders. Employees should ideally follow an organised RTW procedure that entails a number of developing phases and takes into consideration treatment plans, their level of recovery, and employee skills at their point of return when they are returning back to work following a period of sick absence [42]. Nevertheless, due to the complexity that is the

RTW procedure, a percentage of these sick-listed workers frequently undergo a varied and frequently unsatisfactory RTW course, including lengthy or intermittent absence, which has a substantial negative impact on their own well-being as well as that of their employers and society as a whole. Therefore, improper RTW process execution may lead to unexpected RTW results, which may help to explain why agreed-upon RTW measures don't always have the desired effect of helping sick-listed employees. While RTW techniques proved to help certain sick-listed employees in Jetha et al.'s study, negligible results were shown in others. These inconsistent results may indicate that there were variations in the RTW coordinators' competence and the suitability of the agreed-upon RTW plan for employees. It is evident from the above that key RTW players' implementation and skills are a profitable field of research in order to determine the most effective way to help returning workers [68].

The implementation of workplace RTW treatments has been extensively studied, and some writers have proposed that providing suitable modifications or workplace adaptations and dealing with work-related issues are the primary predictors of effective RTW results or job retention. However, there is currently a lack of information about effective workplace-based RTW treatments that outline the accepted RTW techniques, how they operate, and the conditions in which they help people with CMDs or MSDs achieve long-term RTW results. Results from studies by Martimo as well as Viikari-Juntura et al. in particular highlight the challenges involved in simply making adjustments that could lessen the chance of exacerbating an employee's underlying condition. These challenges stem from potential psychosocial, workplace, and management effects [69].

According to some writers, the duration of sick leave may have an effect on whether RTW results for persons with CMDs or MSDs are sustainable. For instance, while examining the relationship between the length of sick leave and RTW results, several writers concentrated on the probability of RTW for patients who were either short- or long-term absentees from work. In these investigations, those classified as short-term absentees (defined as absences lasting less than one week) were shown to have increased sustained RTW compared to people classified as long-term absences (defined as absences lasting more than six weeks). It is unclear, nevertheless, whether the increased sustainable RTW for those categorised as short-term absentees were caused by other reasons or by the applicability of implemented workplace initiatives [45-48].

Western societies' health indicators are becoming better, yet more people are claiming disability and sickness payments for musculoskeletal diseases. Muscular discomfort shouldn't stop you from working or engaging in other activities; doing so will just postpone your recuperation. Therefore, it is obvious that the process of returning to work (RTW) is of great importance for this patient population. It has been extensively studied how acute muscular discomfort leads to chronic illness, missed work, and disability. This research has shown that physical illness, psychological problems, and social variables all affect chronicity and disability. When musculoskeletal discomfort causes more than 8 weeks of absence from work, the prognosis becomes poorer and the likelihood of returning to work decreases [70]

The method of RTW of chronic pain may be seen of as a complicated shift in human behaviour, with the patient ultimately deciding whether or not to undergo RTW. However, the primary entry point for sickness benefits is the general practitioner (GP). Numerous personal, societal, economic, and employment-related aspects affect how the patient perceives their own RTW. A change in conduct is impacted by knowledge, attitudes, norms, and self-efficacy, according to behaviour models [62]. A complex causal structure is proposed by Bandura's Social Cognitive Theory to explain how human motivation, behaviour, and wellbeing are controlled. As regulators of motivation and behaviour in this paradigm, self-efficacy beliefs, objectives, result from expectations, and perceived environmental barriers and facilitators all work in concert. This is in line with the idea that treatments for sick-listed patients with chronic pain should be more centred on coping, managing one's own environmental factors, workplace support, and patient education rather than on treating the underlying pathology. This might improve the patient's expectations for a favourable reaction and result (coping). In accordance with the Cognitive Activation Theories of Stress (CATS), these advancements will reduce the stress response, which might therefore assist patients in treating complaints in a more positive way [63].

As chronic pain should be viewed as multicausal, multidisciplinary treatment (MDA) is generally considered as an acceptable strategy to treating patients. Recent Cochrane reviews indicated that MDA was preferable to conventional treatment in terms of reducing pain and impairment. Multidisciplinary therapies for chronic muscle pain have had contradictory results in terms of their impact on return to work (RTW) [65].

The majority of significant chronic musculoskeletal pain problems, including LBP, are characterised by the absence of objective, pathological findings, despite the fact that patients have diminished work capacity and several additional subjective health concerns. In addition to the patient's explanation of their health, the doctor must also make an effort to comprehend the workplace culture and job requirements in order to make an informed decision about sick leave [66]. Numerous studies have shown the need to increase the number of physicians working in this area, as many general practitioners are hesitant to have workplace conversations with their patients. There is mounting evidence that occupational variables affect disability and that proactive communication from GPs on employment and health initiatives is crucial for RTW. This necessitates strategies in which medical professionals actively evaluate work aspects and health concerns simultaneously during the rehabilitation process [67].

An integrated intervention (MI) is designed to bring attention to the complexity of chronic pain issues. The MI comprised an evaluation of your job, family, lifestyle, coping mechanisms, and health issues. The interdisciplinary Structured Interview with a Visual Teaching Tool (ISIVET) (Figure 21), an innovative teaching tool, was used by the MI to create a visual representation of the patient's condition as a whole. The underlying assumption was that this layout may bring a fresh way of thinking about how to deal with health issues [55]. This might increase patients' willingness to make adjustments, which would improve their ability to cope and return to work. A short intervention programme (BI), based on a non-injury model that has shown to be especially effective on RTW patients with sub-acute LBP, was given to the active control group. The non-injury model relies on the notion that the body and back are sturdy structures, and that pain is not always indicative of harm brought on by improper conduct or other misdeeds [56].

Interventions

The Interview with a Visual Educational Tool (ISIVET) Multidisciplinary Intervention

At first, the patient had separate meetings with the social worker, doctor, and physiotherapist who made up the multidisciplinary team. The patient was initially questioned by the social worker about their family, friends, careers, and finances before working together to determine the working conditions suitable for each individual. This assessed seven distinct factors, including work-related stress, job satisfaction, workload, relationships among coworkers, leadership, level of workplace difficulty, and occupational engagement [58].

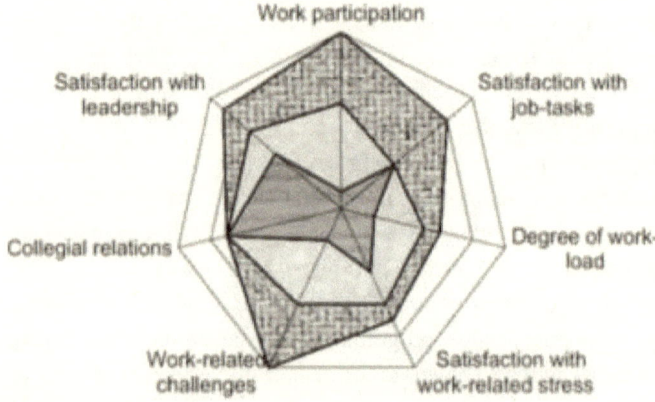

Figure 21: ISIVET's result [58-60]

The patient was initially questioned by the doctor about his or her past and present health as well as that of the family. The doctor then performed a physical examination and came to an ICD-10 diagnosis. Finally, the doctor and the patient worked together to score the "Quality of life" ISIVET-figure. Physical complaints, psychological health, sleep, energy, physical activity, interaction with others, and vocational engagement are all evaluated [59].

The patient's musculoskeletal issues were evaluated by the physiotherapist, who also had a physical examination. 24-Hour Follow-Up For one hour, the patient met with the physiotherapist to discuss the treatment plan and go over the ISIVET once again. A second hue was used to tint the newly created sections. The visualisation of the delta-areas required thought and focus. This served as a reminder of prior counsel and acts, and changes in the rehabilitation plan were finally undertaken [67].

Follow-Up after Three Months For one hour, the patient and the entire team met to summarise the situation and assess the actions made thus far. After completing the ISIVET, fresh spots were coloured using a third hue. They eventually changed the rehabilitative strategy [65]

Four separate doctors whom all had specialties in rehabilitation and physical medicine, and two different social workers, and four different physiotherapists all worked on the MI treatment during the research period [66].

BI, or the Brief Intervention:

The BI consisted of two sessions: an initial appointment lasting about 2.5 hours that included individual consultations with a doctor then a physiotherapist, and then a follow-up appointment with the physiotherapist every two weeks that lasted about an hour [65]. The BI is founded on an LBP non-injury model. It emphasises that the back is a solid and durable structure and that returning to regular exercise would be useful in order to lessen anxiety and enable the patient stay active despite the pain, barring any "red flags" that may be present. The key component of the approach is allowing the patient space and time to communicate their issues, concerns, and ideas. A full medical and educational examination that includes an explanation to the patient of any somatic findings follows [66].

The Hagen handbook and the most recent recommendations served as the foundation for the therapist treatment manuals. The BI was performed by a doctor who specialised in rehabilitation and physical medicine and a physiotherapist. The approach was well-versed by both therapists. 3.5 hours were spent face-to-face addressing the patient throughout the BI [67].

Musculoskeletal discomfort is prolonged by a variety of circumstances. Some are plainly personal to the person, while others are workplace- or compensation-related. Multidisciplinary therapies have shown to be effective in facilitating RTW for low back pain and take into account the fact that barriers to job participation may exist at various levels. Interventions concentrating on these components ought to be of clinical relevance since psychosocial variables predict the long-term disability of musculoskeletal illnesses [68].

References

1. B.P. Bernard Elements of ergonomics programs: a primer based on workplace evaluations of musculoskeletal disorders. US Department of Health and Human Services publication number 97-117.

2. J.T. Albers *et al.* An ergonomic education and evaluation program for apprentice carpenters Am J Ind Med (1997).

3. R.H. Westgaard *et al.* Ergonomic intervention research for improved musculoskeletal health: a critical review Int J Ind Ergon (1997)

4. A. Wisner Variety of physical characteristics in industrially developing countries — ergonomic consequences Int J Ind Ergon (1989)

5. M.C. Haims *et al.* Theory and practice for the implementation of 'in-house', continuous improvement participatory ergonomic programs Appl Ergon (1998)

6. P. Vink *et al.* A participatory ergonomics approach to reduce mental and physical workload Int J Ind Ergonomics (1995)

7. G. Westlander *et al.* Evaluation of an ergonomics intervention program in VDT workplaces Applied Ergonomics (1995)

8. P. Carayon-Sainfort Stress, job control and other job elementsa study of office workers Int J Ind Ergonomic (1991)

9. B. Gardell Autonomy and participation at work Human Relations (1977)

10. M.C. Haims *et al.* Implementation of an in-house participatory ergonomics programa case study in a public service organization

11. M.C. Haims *et al.* Work organization interventions on WRMDs in office/computer work

12. C. Hajnal *et al.* Reflection of a research paradigmthe development and implementation of an ergonomic intervention

13. Ayoub, M. A. (1990). Ergonomic deficiencies: I, pain at work. Journal of Occupational Medicine, 32(1), 52–57.

14. Burri, G. J., and Helander, M. G. (1991). A field study of productivity improvements in the manufacturing of circuit boards. International Journal of Industrial Ergonomics, 7, 207–215.

15. Chapanis, A. (1985). Some reflections on progress. Proceedings of the Human Factors 29th Annual Meeting, Santa Monica, CA, USA, 1–8.

16. Das, B. (1987). An ergonomic approach to designing a manufacturing work system. International Journal of Industrial Ergonomics, 1(3), 231–240.

17. Das, B., and Sengupta, A. (1996). Industrial workstation design: a systematic ergonomic approach. Applied Ergonomics, 27(3), 157–163.

18. Das, B., and Shikdar, A. (1999). Participative versus assigned production standard setting in a repetitive industrial task: a strategy for improving worker productivity. International Journal of Occupational Safety and Ergonomics, 5(3), 417–430.

19. Australian Bureau of Statistics, 2002. Small Business in Australia, 2001. Commonwealth Government, Canberra, Australia.

20. Barrett, J.H., Haslam, R.A., Lee, K.G., Ellis, M.J., 2005. Assessing attitudes and beliefs using the stage of change paradigm - case study of health and safety appraisal within a manufacturing company. Int. J. Industrial Ergonomics 35, 871e887.

21. Bernard, B., 1997. Muscukoskeletal Disorders and Workplace Factors. National Institute for Occupational Safety and Health, Cincinnati, Ohio.

22. Braun, V., Clarke, V., 2006. Using thematic analysis in psychology. Qual. Res. Psychol. 3, 77e101.

23. DeJoy, D.M., 1996. Theoretical models of health behavior and workplace selfprotective behavior. J. Saf. Res. 27, 61e72.

24. Leigh JP, Markowitz SB, Fahs M, Shin C, Landrigan PJ. Occupational Injury and Illness in the United States, Estimates of Costs, Morbidity, and Mortality. Arch Intern Med. 1997; 157(14):1557–68.

25. Palmer KT, Harris EC, Linaker C, Barker M, Lawrence W, Cooper C, et al. Effectiveness of community- and workplace-based interventions to manage musculoskeletal-related sickness absence and job loss: a systematic review. Rheumatology. 2012; 51(2):230–42.

26. United States Department of Labor, Bureau of Labor Statistics. Occupational Injuries and IllnessesAnnual. Nonfatal Occupational Injuries and Illnesses Requiring Days Away From Work. News Releases. (Accessed 19 Nov 2012).

27. Caicoya M, Delclos GL. Work demands and musculoskeletal disorders from the Spanish National Survey. Occup Med. 2010; 60(6):447–50.

28. Kennedy CA, Amick BC, Dennerlien JT, Brewer S, Catli S, William R, et al. Systematic Review of the Role of Occupational Health and Safety Interventions in the Prevention of Upper Extremity Musculoskeletal Symptoms, Signs, Disorders, Injuries, Claims and Lost Time. J Occup Rehabil. 2010; 20(2):127–62.

29. W.C. Allen Overview and Evolution of the ADDIE Training System Adv. Develop. Human Resour., 8 (4) (2006), pp. 430-441, 10.1177/1523422306292942

30. B.C. Amick III, C.C. Menéndez, L. Bazzani, M. Robertson, K. DeRango, T. Rooney, A. Moore

31. A field intervention examining the impact of an office ergonomics training and a highly adjustable chair on visual symptoms in a public sector organization Appl. Ergon., 43 (3) (2012), pp. 625-631, 10.1016/j.apergo.2011.09.006

32. Arksey and O'Malley, 2005 H. Arksey, L. O'Malley Scoping studies: towards a methodological framework Int. J. Soc. Res. Methodol., 8 (1) (2005), pp. 19-32, 10.1080/1364557032000119616

33. Bailey, 2018 Bailey G., 2018. Office workers spend 1,700 hours a year in front of a computer screen. CBC News Los Angeles.

34. Beckmann and Weber, 2016 J. Beckmann, P. Weber Cognitive presence in virtual collaborative learning: Assessing and improving critical thinking in online discussion forums Interactive Technology and Smart Education, 13 (1) (2016), pp. 52-70, 10.1108/ITSE-12-2015-0034

35. Boulos et al., 2014 M.N.K. Boulos, A.C. Brewer, C. Karimkhani, D.B. Buller, R.P. Dellavalle Mobile medical and health apps: state of the art, concerns, regulatory control and certification Online journal of public health informatics, 5 (3) (2014), p. 229, 10.5210/ojphi.v5i3.4814

36. Brewer et al., 2006 S. Brewer, D. Van Eerd, B.C. Amick, E. Irvin, K.M. Daum, F. Gerr, J.S. Moore, K. Cullen, D. Rempel

37. Workplace interventions to prevent musculoskeletal and visu symptoms and disorders among computer users: a systematic review J. Occup. Rehabil., 16 (3) (2006), pp. 325-358, 10.1007/s10926-006-9031-6.

38. Health and Safety Executive (CMDs Report). *Work-Related Stress, Anxiety or Depression Statistics in Great Britain, 2020*; Health and Safety Executive: London, UK, 2020.

39. Health and Safety Executive (MSDs Report). *Work Related Musculoskeletal Disorder Statistics (WRMSDs) in*

Great Britain, 2020; Health and Safety Executive: London, UK, 2020.

40. Hansmann, M.; Beller, J.; Maurer, F.; Kroger, C. Self-Efficacy Beliefs of Employees with Mental Disorders or Musculoskeletal Diseases after Sickness-Related Absence: Validation of the German Version of the Return-to-Work Self-Efficacy Scale. *J. Int. Environ. Res. Public Health* **2022**, *19*, 10093.

41. Health and Safety Executive (HSE). *Mental Health Conditions, Work and the Workplace*; Health and Safety Executive: London, UK, 22 May 2022. Available online: **https://www.hse.gov.uk/stress/mental-health.htm** (accessed on 15 December 2022).

42. World Health Organisation. *Musculoskeletal Health*; World Health Organisation: Geneva, Switzerland, 14 July 2022; Available online: **https://www.who.int/news-room/fact-sheets/detail/musculoskeletal-conditions** (accessed on 15 December 2022).

43. Etuknwa, A.; Daniels, K.; Eib, C. Sustainable Return to Work: A Systematic Review Focusing on Personal and Social Factors. *J. Occup. Rehabil.* **2019**, *29*, 679–700.

44. Lallukka, T.; Hiilamo, A.; Oakman, J.; Manty, M.; Pietilainen, O.; Rahkonen, O.; Kouvonen, A.; Halonen, J.I. Recurrent pain and work disability: A record linkage study. *Int. Arch. Occup. Environ. Health* **2020**, *93*, 421–432.

45. Gaspar, F.W.; Zaidel, C.S.; Dewa, C.S. Rates and predictors of recurrent work disability due to common mental health disorders in the United States. *PLoS ONE* **2018**, *13*, e0205170.

46. Brooks PM. The burden of musculoskeletal disease—a global perspective. Clin Rheumatol. 2006;25(6):778–81.

47. Bevan S, Quadrello T, McGee R, Mahdon M, Vavrovsky A, Barham L. Fit for work. Musculoskeletal disorders in the European workforce. London: The Work Foundation; 2009.

48. Brage S, Ihlebæk C, Natvig B, Bruusgaard D. Muskel-og skjelettlidelser som a°rsak til sykefravær og uføreytelser [Musculoskeletal disorders as causes of sick leave and disability benefits]. Tidsskrift for den Norske laegeforening: tidsskrift for praktisk medicin, ny raekke. 2010;130(23):2369–70.

49. Schultz IZ, Gatchel RJ. Handbook of complex occupational disability claims: early risk identification, intervention, and prevention. Berlin: Springer; 2006.

50. Waddell G, Burton AK. Is work good for your health and wellbeing?. London: The Stationery Office; 2006.

51. Gross AR, Goldsmith C, Hoving JL, Haines T, Peloso P, Aker P, et al. Conservative management of mechanical neck disorders: a systematic review. J Rheumatol. 2007;34(5):1083–102.

52. Koes BW, van Tulder M, Lin CWC, Macedo LG, McAuley J, Maher C. An updated overview of clinical guidelines for the management of non-specific low back pain in primary care. Eur Spine J. 2010;19(12):2075–94.

53. Waddell G, Burton AK. Occupational health guidelines for the management of low back pain at work: evidence review. Occup Med. 2001;51(2):124–35.

54. Hagen KB, Thune O. Work incapacity from low back pain in the general population. Spine. 1998;23(19):2091–5.

55. Burton AK, Tillotson KM, Main CJ, Hollis S. Psychosocial predictors of outcome in acute and subchronic low back trouble. Spine. 1995;20(6):722–8.

56. Bendix AF, Bendix T, Hæstrup C. Can it be predicted which patients with chronic low back pain should be offered tertiary rehabilitation in a functional restoration program? A search for demographic, socioeconomic, and physical predictors. Spine. 1998;23(16):1775–83.

57. Brage S, Kann I. Fastlegers sykmeldingspraksis I: Variasjoner [General practitioners' sickness certification practices]. Report. 2006;6:1–38.

58. Krause N, Dasinger LK, Deegan LJ, Rudolph L, Brand RJ. Psychosocial job factors and return-to-work after compensated low back injury: a disability phase-specific analysis. Am J Ind Med. 2001;40(4):374–92.

59. Schultz I, Stowell A, Feuerstein M, Gatchel R. Models of return to work for musculoskeletal disorders. J Occup Rehabil. 2007;17(2):327–52.

60. Franche R-L, Krause N. Readiness for return to work following injury or illness: conceptualizing the interpersonal impact of health care, workplace, and insurance factors. J Occup Rehabil. 2002;12(4):233–56.

61. Ajzen I. The theory of planned behavior. Organ Behav Hum Decis Process. 1991;50(2):179–211.

62. United States Department of Labor, Bureau of Labor Statistics *Occupational Injuries and Illnesses-Annual. Nonfatal*

Occupational Injuries and Illnesses Requiring Days Away From Work. News Releases. (Accessed 19 Nov 2012).

63. Caicoya M, Delclos GL. Work demands and musculoskeletal disorders from the Spanish National Survey. *Occup Med.* 2010;60(6):447–50.

64. Kennedy CA, Amick BC, Dennerlien JT, Brewer S, Catli S, William R, et al. Systematic Review of the Role of Occupational Health and Safety Interventions in the Prevention of Upper Extremity Musculoskeletal Symptoms, Signs, Disorders, Injuries, Claims and Lost Time. *J Occup Rehabil.* 2010;20(2):127–62.

65. National Research Council and Institute of Medicine. *Musculoskeletal Disorders and the Workplace: Low Back and Upper Extremities.* The National Academy Press; Washington, DC: 2001. pp. 364–5.

66. Valachi K, Valachi B. Mechanisms leading to musculosketetal disorders in dentistry. JADA 2003;10:1344-50.

67. Saunders H, Saunders R. Evaluations, treatment and prevention of musculoskeletal disorders. Vol. 1. Chaska, Minn.: Educational Opportunities; 1995:7.

68. Norkin C, Levangie P. Joint structure and function: A comprehensive analysis. 2nd ed. Philadelphia: F.A. Davis; 1992:126-8.

69. Hertling D, Kessler R. Management of common musculoskeletal disorders: Physical therapy principles and methods. 3rd ed. Philadelphia: Lippincott; 1996:551-2.

70. Hagberg M. ABC of work related disorders: neck and arm disorders. BMJ 1996;313(7054):419-22.

71. Hedman T, Fernie G. Mechanical response of the lumbar spine to seated postural loads. Spine 1997;22:734-43.

Chapter 5:

Legal And Ethical Considerations

Introduction

Concerns about the moral and legal issues surrounding the conduct of clinical research involving human subjects have long been voiced by policymakers, attorneys, scientists, and doctors. Clinical research seeks to improve clinical practice and help patients in the future by methodically gathering and analyzing data from which generalizable conclusions can be made. To ensure that the research is carried out both ethically and legally, it is crucial to be familiar with Good Clinical Practice (GCP), an international quality standard offered by the International Conference on Harmonisation (ICH) of Technical Requirements for Registration of Pharmaceuticals for Human Use, or the local version, GCP of the Central Drugs Standard Control Organisation [1]. Because of how aging affects society, chronic disease has grown to be a significant burden on an already overburdened healthcare system. The fact that many illnesses of this type may coexist in the same person compounds their effects. More than a quarter of adults, according to current prevalence estimates, have numerous chronic diseases, and 14% of Medicare beneficiaries have six or more. The US Department of Health and Human Services (HHS) has published a report on this issue in recognition of the systemic stresses now present, such as the aging population and rising healthcare costs. The "Strategic Framework on

Multiple Chronic Conditions" is the first formal attempt to define the broad challenges presented by these conditions, such as the need for improved home- and community-based programs as well as improved management of medications, and to provide a framework for improving the health status of people with multiple chronic conditions [2].

Musculoskeletal diseases are the number one cause of disability in the United States as well as more than half of the total chronic illnesses in adults over 50 in industrialised countries. These disorders, which are more common than other more well-known ailments like heart disease, diabetes, and cancer despite not often being a cause of mortality, impact younger populations of all genders and races, and are a significant cause of pain, and lower quality of life [2]. When taken as a whole, the incidence of musculoskeletal illnesses is really only surpassed by chronic hypertension and lipid metabolic disorders. Lower back pain was the most prevalent musculoskeletal ailment, with approximately 60 million persons reporting it on a regular basis. Neck discomfort and aching joints, such as those associated with rheumatic and connective tissue illnesses, are additional serious problems [1-3].

Chronic illness, the health care system, and morality

Examples of musculoskeletal disorders include osteoarthritis, connective tissue diseases like scleroderma and systemic lupus erythematosus, inflammatory diseases like rheumatoid arthritis, and problems of the spine. These chronic musculoskeletal illnesses can frequently be controlled with current therapy, but they are typically incurable and reduce the quality of life owing to pain and/or movement restrictions [3]. Even though the sufferer's life is frequently interrupted by concurrent, severe illnesses that require immediate medical attention, a great deal of the patient's care is typically provided outside of hospitals, with frequent doctor visits and a reliance on others to help with daily activities. The poor, minorities and the destitute are disproportionately affected, along with other already marginalised elements of our society [4].

Because of how ageing affects society, chronic illness has grown to be a significant burden on an already overburdened healthcare system. The fact that many illnesses of this type can occur in the same person compounds their effects. More than a quarter of individuals, according to recent prevalence estimates, have numerous chronic illnesses, and 14% of Medicare recipients have six or more [5]. The US Department for Health and Human Services, or HHS, has published a paper about this issue after realising the system's current pressures, such as the ageing population and growing healthcare costs. The "Strategic Framework in Multiple Chronic Conditions" is the first formal attempt to define the broad difficulties posed by these conditions, including the need for improved home- as well as community-based services and enhancing medication management, and to provide a framework for enhancing the health status of people with multiple chronic conditions [6].

Despite the fact that more individuals are becoming afflicted by these problems, the public and the healthcare system give chronic diseases less attention and assistance than they do acute illnesses. Well-known catchphrases imply a focus against cure rather than an approach that emphasises care, such as the "war on cancer," the "race to a cure," or "strike out MS." [7].

Disability Law

Disability is frequently an unavoidable result of chronic rheumatic and musculoskeletal illness because of the pain and functional limitations it causes. As a result, it is important to recognise the ethical aspects of the disability problem, which will be covered in further detail in Dr. Goering's article that is part of this series. Here, a few opening remarks are provided [3,5].

On a historical point, it wasn't till the nineteenth century when scientific studies classified differences in human shape and functioning as a category of abnormality and deviance that the term "disability" came into being. This viewpoint has evolved significantly through time, much as the ailments that are considered to be incapacitating. The range of illnesses that are now regarded as impairments is broad, and it includes anything from paraplegia, blindness, and even autism to multiple sclerosis, the loss of a limb, and psychiatric problems. Chronic rheumatic as well as musculoskeletal illnesses are at the forefront of them [6].

From a philosophical perspective, there are two conflicting theories that define disability. The medical model views impairments considered a condition that may be treated or repaired and as a normal, unavoidable result of a disease process that typically affects a bodily component. The social model, in contrast, attributes the negative aspects of disability to social variables, particularly the hostile environment that a person with a disability must live in. Therefore, the framework used to treat disability substantially determines the perception of how such problems may be addressed based on how one views the impact of impairment on well-being [5].

Occupational Health and Safety Regulations

All non-government companies are required under the Occupational Health and Safety Act of 1970 to maintain a secure and healthy work environment for their staff. It also allowed for the establishment of the National Institute of Occupational Health and Safety (NIOSH) and the Occupational Safety and Health Administration (OSHA). The statute mandates that OSHA create and publish standards using a transparent rule-making procedure. Employers are required to adhere to these OHS guidelines just as they would any other legal obligation [8].

The OSHA standard 29 CFR Section 1910 is where you'll find the most significant federal regulations pertaining to OHS. Numerous aspects of the text are relevant to the work done in settings wherein nonhuman primates are utilised for research, instruction, and testing [9].

For instance, the Occupational Safety and Health Administration's bloodborne pathogens standard mandates that institutions give hepatitis B vaccinations to staff who handle blood, organs, and other tissues to experimental animals infected with the hepatitis B virus. Additionally, institutions must provide the staff with a private medical evaluation as soon as they have contact with animal tissues that have been contaminated with a bloodborne pathogen. When monitoring reveals an amount of exposure that frequently surpasses the threshold for action for an OSHA-regulated substance, like a time-weighted typical of 0.75 ppm or a short-term contact of 2.0 ppm over formaldehyde (29 CFR 1910.1048), the OSHA standard on occupational contact with hazardous chemicals within laboratories calls for medical surveillance [1,5].

The OSHA standard governing the consumption of gases that are compressed is 29 CFR 1910.101, the standards for personal protective equipment, or PPE, are 29 CFR 1910.132-1910.140, and the regulations for electric systems are 29 CFR 1910.301-1910.330, however other portions of 29 CFR 1910 may also be relevant [6].

It's crucial to remember that the OSHA regulations don't cover everything. They don't immediately address each danger or hazard that exists at every workplace. The general duty clause of the Act on Occupational Safety and Health, which requires employers to provide workplaces "free from recognised hazards which are causing or are probable to cause death and serious physical harm," may be used by OSHA to address hazards that are not covered by a specific standard [9].

Office of Health and Safety at Work

The government organisation OSHA is in charge of safeguarding workers' health and avoiding occupational illnesses, fatalities, and injuries. Despite the fact that OSHA and NIOSH were established by the same congressional legislation, they are independent organisations with distinct missions. Regulations pertaining to occupational health and safety must be developed and implemented by OSHA. By means of inspections and financial penalties, it creates protective occupational norms and enforces them. Additionally, it offers free on-site assistance in identifying and eliminating dangers as well as help set up OHS programmes [10].

The Occupational Health and Safety National Institute (NIOSH)

The government organisation NIOSH is in charge of conducting studies and formulating suggestions for preventing illnesses and accidents at work. Together, NIOSH and OSHA frequently collaborate to safeguard the health and safety of employees [11].

NIOSH is a great resource for both organisations and people looking for information about OHS. It publishes hazard-specific guidelines (also known as "hazard IDs"), including Cercopithecine herpesvirus 1 (B Virus) An infection Resulting to Ocular Exposure, which can be found and offers a summary of the most important details, a description of the hazard, suggestions for avoiding B virus infections, suggested actions, and references for more information [11].

Employee obligations and rights

As a worker, an individual is subjected to access and exercise the following rights [11-12]:

1. A healthy and safe workplace

2. Any details your company may have on any possible contact you may have encountered with dangers like loud noises or dangerous substances. Additionally, you are entitled to any medical files that your employer may hold about you.

3. to request that the company address hazardous situations.

4. to take part in inspections for enforcement.

5. to be protected from prejudice if you exercise your right to health and safety. If you exercise your right to health and safety, your employer cannot dismiss you, intimidate you, insult you, or conduct you differently.

6. should decline tasks that might put you in immediate risk of injury. Request that the company remove the risk before stating that you will take an alternative assignment from their company. The OSHA law only offers protection if the risk can be established; if you decline a job because you think a condition is dangerous but are later shown to be mistaken, OSHA does not offer such protection.

7. You have access to information about the risks at work, the chemicals used there, the measurements of chemical, noise, and radiation levels your company has made, as well as what to do if an accident occurs or if you or other workers are exposed to other dangerous substances.

8. to give information to your employer on OSHA requirements, work-related illnesses and injuries, safety risks, and employee rights [12].

You should receive training on the substances you are subjected to at work from your employer, along with instructions on how to be safe. On additional health and safety risks and requirements that the company you work for must adhere to.

It is your duty as an employee to:

1. Read the job site's health and safety at work poster.

2. Follow all relevant OSHA and Maine safety regulations.

3. Wear or make use of the necessary protective equipment while working, and adhere to all legal employer safety and health laws and regulations.

4. Inform the company of any dangerous circumstances.

5. Inform the manager of any illness or injury that occurred on the work, and get help right away.

6. employers' obligations

7. Employers are required to follow the Occupational Health and Safety Act of 1970 as well as Maine law [13].

Establish a workplace without dangerous risks

1. Observe OSHA regulations

2. Ensure that workers are using and possessing safe equipment and tools. Maintain this equipment as it should be.

3. Use labels, signs, posters, or colour codes to alert staff to possible dangers.

4. Establish or revise operational guidelines and disseminate them to ensure that staff adheres to safety and health regulations.

5. When OSHA regulations call for it, give medical exams and instructions. The OSHA poster and the State of Maine Occupational Health and Safety poster alerting workers to their rights and obligations should be displayed where employees may see it (public sector employers) [14].

Immediately report fatalities and hospitalisations:

1. Private Sector: Any accident that results in a fatality or three or more hospitalised personnel must be reported to a local OSHA office (780-3178) within eight hours.

2. Maine Public Sector: within 24 hours if a wounded employee requires an overnight hospital stay, and within 8 hours in the event of a fatality, to the Bureau of Labour Standards Workplace Health and Safety Division.

3. Keep track of any illnesses or injuries sustained at work and post those data. Employers in some low-hazard businesses and those in the private sector with less than 10 employees are free from this obligation.

4. Access to the Work-Related Injuries and Illnesses Log should be made available to current and past employees as well as their representatives.

5. Provide employees or their authorised representatives with access to medical and exposure records.

6. Not to treat workers unfairly who assert their rights to safety and health.

7. Post citations near or adjacent to the affected work location. Each citation shall stay displayed for the greater of

three working days or until the infraction has been remedied. documentation or tags used to verify post-abatement work.

8. Correct identified violations by the time specified in the citation, and submit the necessary documents for abatement verification [15].

Ethical Considerations in Managing MSDs

Many new issues have emerged in recent years as a result of changes in the workplace, fragmentation, economic challenges, demographic changes, new technology, and, more broadly, the effects of globalisation. With an increase in the percentage of women, immigrants, and older workers in the workforce, it is also becoming more diverse. A growing body of research on the effects of new work organisation structures—such as modifications to management practices, the use of contractors as well as temporary workers, adjustments to working hours, and increased flexibility to work from home or elsewhere—has highlighted detrimental effects on workers' health and safety. Workplace management can impact how much psychological stress employees feel and exacerbate existing health issues (eg. diabetes, metabolic syndrome, cardiovascular disease, and musculoskeletal diseases) relating to the possibility of getting hurt or ill from exposure to workplace dangers [16].

These demand fundamental changes in occupational health, which is seen as a key component of the social dimension of working life, in line with a more expansive concept of global and integrated promotion of well-being at work, posing a number of new challenges for employees and their representatives, employers, managers, health service providers, government authorities, professional associations, and social partners [16].

The traditional focus on "health risk management" has been expanded by a new paradigm in occupational health to encompass workplace health promotion, support for chronic non-communicable diseases, and treatment of these conditions, in addition to the medical components of sick leave and rehabilitation. The overlap between the two realms of "prevention" (of dangers) and "promotion" (of health) has grown during the last few decades. Currently, "occupational health" is designed to encompass both workplace health promotion and health protection [15].

Due to their increasingly complex and sometimes conflicting obligations to employees, employers, the general public, public health and labour authorities, and other organisations like social security and judicial authorities, occupational health professionals (OHPs) play a crucial role in this scenario. The ability to operate as a care provider, an expert, a decision-maker, a communicator and a counselor, a leader and an advisor, and a manager will become increasingly important for occupational physicians in the future years. A reassessment of the OHPs' competency and capacity will be necessary in light of new difficulties and working methods, with implications for the health and safety of future employees [13,14].

All individuals who do occupational health and safety-related duties, offer occupational health services, or engage in occupational health practises are referred to as OHPs in this context. OHPs are therefore those who conduct occupational health and safety research as well as occupational health physicians, occupational health nurses, factory inspectors, occupational hygienists, occupational psychologists, ergonomists, specialists in rehabilitation therapy, accident prevention, and the improvement of the working environment [15].

In terms of their duties (such as health surveillance, workplace monitoring, interventions to prevent health hazards, employee ability assessments, pre-employment health examinations, risk assessments, rehabilitation of workers with health disorders, etc.) and professional behaviour, OHPs will be operating within new contexts as a result of this scenario. The repercussions of a health professional's concurrent commitments, whether explicit or implicit, to a third party could have a negative effect on a patient, client, or client community [17].

Particularly, in recent years, there has been an increase in regulatory complexity, emerging concerns about diagnostic tests that may be unethical or technological innovation, increasing the complexity of the decision-making process, and emphasising the role of health professionals in balancing the interests of individuals (i.e., the health and working capacity of individual employees), the enterprise (i.e., maximising production), and the public good [18].

However, due to an increase in potential stakeholders, the ethical decision has grown even more complex and heterogeneous in the age of globalisation, taking into account history, culture, religion, value systems, and social practises. Examples include the conflict between a worker's right to life, health, and safety and a company's right to maximise productivity, or between a worker's right to risk disclosure and a company's right to industrial secrecy, as well as the rights and obligations of OHPs. Another significant development in occupational health is the emergence of a multidisciplinary approach (technical, medical, social, and legal), which denotes the inclusion of additional specialists from different professions in occupational health services [19].

Rehabilitation and Disability Management

The following are a few conditions that could benefit from musculoskeletal rehab:

- Amputation

- Achilles tendon injuries and shoulder rotator cuff tears are two examples of tendon damage

- Trauma injuries, including fractures, joint dislocations, sprains, and strains

- backache

- Osteoporosis

- Arthritis

- Bone cancer

- ailments brought on by repeated stress, including tendonitis and carpal tunnel syndrome

- Joint replacement after injury

Programmes for musculoskeletal rehabilitation can be completed either in inpatient department or outpatient department. The rehabilitation team includes several qualified individuals, including the following:

- orthopaedic surgeons and orthopedists

- Neurologist/neurosurgeon

- Physiatrist

- Internist

- Other medical specialists

- Rehabilitation professionals

- licensed nutritionist

- bodily therapist

- Workplace therapist

- the social worker

- Physiologist of exercise

- Psychologist/psychiatrist

- Therapies for recreation

- the case manager

- Chaplain

- a career counsellor

Individual state workers' compensation programmes spend upwards of $3 billion annually on musculoskeletal injuries to the hand and wrist, shoulder, cervical spine, lumbar spine, and knee. The average medical costs per lost-time claim have been estimated at 29000 US dollars. WRMSDs can cause significant personal financial hardship and family disruption in addition to the significant societal impact. The negative effects of WRMSDs are particularly evident for patients who reach a plateau in their targeted outpatient treatment but still experience persistent physical or medical issues or other constraints that prevent them from returning to work. These persons experience prolonged absences from the workforce, sometimes lasting years, and are frequently referred to vocational rehabilitation programmes for further care [19,20].

Occupational rehabilitation programmes are post-acute, comprehensive therapy interventions with goals of improving physical capacities, enhancing client safety, and addressing psychological outcomes for people with work-related injuries so that they can tolerate a return to gainful employment [18,19]. Programmes for occupational rehabilitation use a multimodal or multidisciplinary approach, or both, to deliver therapy to improve overall tolerance levels for work demands. Patients are typically referred for treatment of a physical ailment, but occupational rehabilitation programmes also help to enhance psychological variables and quality of life [20].

To determine the client and programme characteristics that enhance return-to-work results in occupational rehabilitation programmes, numerous research studies have been conducted. The severity of symptomatology, type of injury, time since injury, age and gender, as well as the physical demands of the profession, are some of the important factors that have come to light [20].

Occupational Rehabilitation Programs

The clinic offered work conditioning and work hardening as general and comprehensive occupational rehabilitation programs, respectively. The main objective of the general occupational rehabilitation programme, which was offered by one discipline (for example, occupational therapy), was to increase the general physical tolerance and endurance needed for a client to successfully return to part-time employment, which is defined as up to 20 hours per week. The comprehensive occupational rehabilitation programme, in contrast, was a specially designed plan offered to patients with complex cases who needed interdisciplinary care (such as occupational therapy, physical therapy, psychology, dietetics, and nursing) and individualised, intensive rehabilitation to increase tolerance for going back to full-time employment at a 40-hour workweek. Over the course of the nine-year data collection period, the same occupational therapist oversaw both programmes. The comprehensive programme typically began with participants at a higher duration and frequency with the aim of progressing to a maximum of 8 hr, 5 days/week. In contrast, the general programme was initiated at a minimum session duration of 2 hr, 3 days/week, and progressed to a maximum of 4-5 hr, 5 days/week, as tolerated [18,19].

A progressive whole-body flexibility routine, cardiovascular endurance training, strengthening exercises, core stability training, and general job simulation (i.e., occupation-based activities) were the five main components of both programmes. Although the basic elements of both programmes were the same, the activities varied based on the program's objectives [20].

Depending on the skills of each client, the quantity, length, repetition, and frequency of activities within each component were regularly increased. Clients in the comprehensive programme also received counseling from a psychologist, took part in hour-long educational seminars (such as those on stress management and thorough body mechanics training), and had consultations with other team members as needed (such as those on diet and medication management) [20].

Primary Outcome

Return to work is the ideal result for treating job-related injuries, but many of the clients who were referred to this institution had been out of work for several months or even years by the time they arrived, making an immediate return to work option impossible. As a result, the main finding of this study dissociated actual return to work from appropriate physical capacity gains indicating readiness for gainful employment. As a result, the main indicator of success was when clients were discharged and met one or more of the following three requirements: (1) returned to work at any job, (2) were given the all-clear by a doctor to return to work and started looking for a job, or (3) advanced to additional services as part of a vocational rehabilitation plan designed to support finding employment. A client was deemed unsuccessful if any one of the following three circumstances occurred: (1) increased medical needs necessitating a higher level of care; (2) early retirement; (3) dropping out of the programme; or (4) inability to tolerate sustained activities necessary for part-time work [20].

Practitioners of occupational therapy are specially trained to concentrate on occupation in all of its forms. Practitioners should incorporate occupation-based techniques into their interventions rather than only using them as part of the evaluation process (AOTA, 2014; Gillen, 2013). Work-related rehabilitation is a natural fit for occupational therapy practitioners given the importance of the occupation of work as a life role and its contribution to people's meaning and purpose. The use of work-related occupation-based activities deserves more investigation while being frequently overshadowed by a focus on daily living activities within physical rehabilitation research [17].

The following specific suggestions for practise and research:

• Occupational therapy practitioners should offer an intensive, multicomponent rehabilitation programme that supports recovery for people with WRMSDs who are unable to return to work after receiving traditional, injury-focused therapy services.

• Participation in simulated work activities is a strong predictor of successful occupational rehabilitation and supports the need to use an occupational perspective not on injury.

• The level of therapeutic engagement is a crucial factor in the success of occupational rehabilitation programmes, so participants in these programmes should be allowed to increase the number of weekly sessions and the number of hours per session as tolerated.

• To fully grasp the intricacies of predictors for success in occupational rehabilitation, more extensive prospective research and qualitative evaluation of client success are required [21].

Autonomy

Autonomous decision-making in chronic disease is more challenging compared to acute treatment, when ethical dilemmas typically result from disputes, are constrained in scope and length, and are typically resolved by the patient and their doctor. The ethical conundrums that arise in the context of chronic diseases take on more emotional and social as well as medical aspects, may call for the participation of several parties, and, if they do, take longer to resolve [21].

Agich is aware that difficulties brought on by chronic illnesses are frequently less spectacular and involve fewer conflicts than those brought on by acute illnesses. Accordingly, he argues that decision-making in chronic illness requires a different strategy than it does in acute care. He makes a distinction between decisions that are typically considered to be difficult in the literature on medical ethics and those that patients perceive to be difficult [20,21]. He refers to the first category of decisions as nodal decisions, and they occur when there are distinct alternatives, costs, and benefits that must be assessed, and coercion may be involved due to power imbalances between the participants. He also focuses on other decisions, which he refers to as interstitial decisions because they take place in situations that are thought of as routine. These implicit decisions are made rather than made overtly, and frequently one may arrive at them without being conscious that active consideration is necessary to make the decisions. Although humans value making both of these kinds of judgments, the relevance of interstitial decision-making has been overshadowed by the focus that medical professionals and ethicists have placed on nodal-type decisions [19-21].

Agich argues that an effective definition of autonomy must be understood in terms of the entirety of options and relationships in order to account for the importance of these various decision-making processes. Therefore, he makes a distinction between ideal and actual autonomy. Ideal autonomy is the capacity of individuals to act as rational, independent decision-makers who are aware of their own desires. Ideal autonomy is abstract, cut off from the real world and from what people actually do in it. In contrast, real autonomy is much more diverse than ideal autonomy. It has to do with the unique reality of the individual making the choice. It draws on real-world experience and concentrates on the reality faced by the person making the decision [14].

These ideas of true autonomy and decision-making match the circumstances of the chronically ill better. Nodal-type decisions or ideal autonomy are not, of course, irrelevant when it comes to caring for people with chronic conditions. But in this situation, patients may find that those choices are less important and pertinent than the daily choices they make, and the worries about whether they will be able to carry on with those choices. As a result, when caring for patients with chronic illnesses, medical professionals must consider how to improve their autonomy and capacity for making decisions. The options presented and selections made have to be an accurate reflection of the person as a unique being with a certain past and set of values [22].

Occupational Safety, Health and Working Condition Code, 2019 (Ministry of Labour and Employment, Government of India

Context

The terms of labor laws are protected by the Concurrent List of the Constitution. The Code consolidates 13 Acts regulating workers' health safety and working conditions. Basically, this law covers labours, construction workers, employees, journalists and other occupations. Even different acts cover establishments based on various thresholds of workers such as factories, motor transport, contract labour and more.

Key Features

Coverage and Registration:

- Applies to establishments with 10 or more workers, including all mines and docks.

- Mandatory registration for covered establishments.

- Factories require an additional license, and contractors hiring 20 or more workers can obtain a 5-year license. Beedi workers' license validity extended from 1 to 3 years.

Authorities:

- Inspectors-cum-facilitators empowered to conduct inspections and investigate accidents.

- Occupational Safety and Health Advisory Boards at national and state levels to advise governments on rule formulation.

Duties of Employers:

- Provide a hazard-free workplace, issue appointment letters, and ensure risk-free conditions for employees.

- Additional duties in specific sectors (factories, mines, docks, plantations, construction) include providing a safe workplace and employee training.

- Contract labor employers obligated to provide welfare facilities.

Work Hours and Leave:

- Limit of 6 working days per week for all workers, with exceptions for motor transport workers.

- Government-set maximum working hours for establishments.

- Paid annual leave entitlement of at least 1 in 20 days of duty.

- Overtime work eligible for twice the wage.

- Working journalists restricted to 144 hours in four weeks.

- Sales promotion employees entitled to earned leave and medical leave based on time spent on duty.

Health and Welfare Facilities:

- Working conditions, including a hygienic environment, clean water, and toilets, to be notified by the central government.

- Additional welfare facilities such as canteens, first aid boxes, and creches may be prescribed.

Special Provisions:

- Female workers, with consent, are permitted to work beyond 7 pm and before 6 am.

- Prohibition of children below 14 years from employment.

References

1. The burden of musculoskeletal disease in the United States, 2008. www.boneandjointburden.org.

2. Medical Expenditure Panel Survey. 2004. www.ahrq.gov/about/ cj2004/meps04 htm.

3. Gibson J, Upshur R. Ethics and chronic disease: where are the bioethicists? Bioethics. 2012;26(5):ii–v.

4. Parekh AK, Kronick R, Tavenner M. Optimizing health for persons with multiple chronic conditions. JAMA. 2014;312(12):1199–200.

5. Parekh AK, Goodman RA, Gordon C, HSS Interagency Workgroup on Multiple Chronic Conditions, et al. Managing multiple chronic conditions: a strategic framework for improving health outcomes and quality of life. Public Health Rep. 2010;126(4):460–71.

6. Callahan D. When self-determination runs amok. Hast Cent Rep. 1992;22(2):52–5.

7. Beauchamp TL, Childress JF. Principles of biomedical ethics. 6th ed. New York: Oxford University Press; 2009.

8. National Research Council (US) Committee on Occupational Health and Safety in the Care and Use of Nonhuman Primates. Occupational Health and Safety in the Care and Use of Nonhuman Primates. Washington (DC): National Academies Press (US); 2003. 6, Occupational Health and Safety Regulations and Recommendations Applicable to Nonhuman-Primate Research Facilities. Available from: https://www.ncbi.nlm.nih.gov/books/NBK43453/

9. Iavicoli, S., Valenti, A., Gagliardi, D., and Rantanen, J. (2018). Ethics and Occupational Health in the Contemporary World of Work. *International Journal of Environmental Research and Public Health, 15*(8).

10. ILO . *Changing Patterns in the World of Work.* ILO; Geneva, Switzerland: 2006. [(accessed on 28 March 2018)]. International Labour Conference 95th Session 2006, Report I (C) Available online: http://www.ilo.org/public/english/standards/relm/ilc/ilc95/pdf/rep-i-c.pdf

11. Ronchetti M., Di Tecco C., Russo S., Castaldi T., Vitali S., Autieri S., Valenti A., Persechino B., Iavicoli S. An integrated approach to the assessment of work-related stress risk: Comparison of findings from two tools in an Italian methodology. *Saf. Sci.* 2015;**80**:310–316. doi: 10.1016/j.ssci.2015.08.005.

12. ILO . *Emerging Risks and New Patterns of Prevention in a Changing World of Work—World Day for Safety and Health at Work 28 April 2010.* ILO; Geneva, Switzerland: 2010.

13. Iavicoli S. The new EU occupational safety and health strategic framework 2014–2020: Objectives and challenges. *Occup. Med. (Lond.)* 2016;**66**:180–182. doi: 10.1093/occmed/kqw010.

14. Harrison J., Dawson L. Occupational Health: Meeting the Challenges of the Next 20 Years. *Saf. Health Work.* 2016;7:143–149. doi: 10.1016/j.shaw.2015.12.004.

15. Franco G. The role of the occupational physician in the enlarged European Union: Challenges and opportunities. *Occup. Med.* 2006;**3**:152–154. doi: 10.1093/occmed/kqj017.

16. Berlinguer G. La medicina del lavoro all'inizio del secolo XX. Riflessioni sul I Congresso Internazionale (1906) e sul I Congresso Nazionale (1907) per le malattie da lavoro. In: Grieco A., Bertazzi P.A., editors. *Per una Storiografia Italiana della Prevenzione Occupazionale ed Ambientale.* Franco Angeli; Milano, Italy: 1997.

17. Franco G. Virtù e valori etici della Diatriba. Un tributo a Bernardino Ramazzini in occasione del trecentesimo anniversario della morte (1714) *Med. Lav.* 2014;**105**:3–14.

18. Smith A. *An Inquiry into the Nature and Causes of the Wealth of Nations.* 5th ed. Methuen and Co., Ltd; London, UK:

1904. [(accessed on 20 September 2016)]. Available online: http://www.econlib.org/library/Smith/smWN.html

19. De Gasperi A. *I tempi e gli uomini che Prepararono la "Rerum novarum".* Vita e Pensiero; Milano, Italy: 1931.

20. Franco G. *Meglio prevenire che curare. Il pensiero di Bernardino Ramazzini medico sociale e scienziato visionario.* Narcissus (Epub); Loreto, Ancona, Italy: 2015.

21. Global Ethic Foundation . *Global Economic Ethics—Consequences for Global Business.* Global Ethic Foundation; Tuebingen, Germany: 2009. A Manifesto Published by the Global Ethic Foundation.

22. Avishai M. In: *The Decent Society.* Goldblum N., translator. Harvard University Press; London, UK: 1998.

www.ingramcontent.com/pod-product-compliance
Lightning Source LLC
LaVergne TN
LVHW091626070526
838199LV00044B/962